# Re-Run

My 30 day Experiment to Fall Back in Love with Running

Tony Markey

*Tony Markey*

# Contents

# ACKNOWLEDGMENTS

Dedicated to my wife Denise, from whom all my running inspiration comes. It's not quite sufficient to say she's my inspiration, because I was so out of love with running for so long there would have been no running without her. I'd probably be eating chips on a literal couch somewhere, not running and not caring about it, were it not for her personal commitment to running. So her commitment to herself was my inspiration. I'm so inspired that I wrote this poem to you, darling:

You make the inspiration.
I make the perspiration.
Let's get sweaty together.

Is that a haiku? Seems like a haiku. At least it's haiku-like.

I also want to thank my children, without whom I would not be a Dad.

Kudos to my main homeslice, Zorro. The REAL one. No, not Antonio Banderas. No, that black and white show was okay, but no. George Hamilton? What? NO. Alain Delon, the only real Zorro. Well it's not my fault you don't know that one. Well now you'll have to go google that, won't you.

Seriously, thanks to all my family that supported me through this process, and to the readers too, because readers help people make the distinction between author and weird old guy with axe to grind or nonsense to spew.

Also, thanks to Running, without which there would be no book. It'd be a series of bad, nonsensical jokes referring to a nonexistent activity, and that would be really weird. A lot like this acknowledgements section..

# PROLOGUE: HOW I CAME TO HATE RUNNING

I was a youthful Zephyr, flying with the wind in my face, fleet of foot and bold of spirit. I was the fastest boy in my 5th grade class, and it seemed like I could run anywhere, at any speed I chose. If I wanted to get there sooner I would just run faster. Running was second nature. I was epic and awesome.

You might ask: "Why did you run everywhere?" If you asked me then, I would have said: "Why would you walk anywhere?"

But 35 years later I have a sorrowful confession to make.

I hate running.

*Sobbing*

Actually, "hate" may be too weak a word. I have some of the same feelings about running as I do about death: it's going to happen. It's going to suck. And after it happens, I will probably end up in a pine box.

How did running fall from grace in my mind? How did a kid who ran everywhere turn into a grumpy middle aged man who views his two to three runs per week(fine, okay, one or two.) as such a danged chore? Wheeeeeeeze.

It may have started in the sixth grade when I discovered biking. In fact, biking replaced running and I biked everywhere, even riding three miles to soccer practice and three miles home afterwards.

For a sixth grader, running was to biking what cars were to rockets: too slow. Too little so see. Too mundane. Biking was cheap transport, too, and became more of a necessity as I neared driving age with no car and no means to see friends other than hopping on a bike and riding at least a couple of miles.

Oh sure, I could have run. But when was the last time you jogged to work instead of hopping in the car? Exactly.

Running lost some of its allure, though I was still fairly fast and I definitely enjoyed it. I ran track briefly in High School, and though I never finished better than fifth in any event(okay, full disclosure. There were sometimes 5 runners), I felt every bit a runner. Crazily, I even ran in -40 degree weather in my hometown of Fairbanks, Alaska, putting a garbage bag over a shirt and my track sweatshirt over both, wearing a scarf over my mouth to ward against the cold air.

I was a teenage running idiot. Clearly.

In college I joined the National Guard and in my advanced training(AIT) I ran the two-mile in 12:30. I had never run faster before or since. I was pretty quick, and proud of it. If you have run faster than that, I would love to talk about it. We could sit down and discuss it over a beer and then I could poke you in the eye.

That was pretty much the end of running for awhile. I played intramural football and a little rugby in college, - who needs brain cells? - but after college running was pretty much a once-every-few-months-maybe affair. I had work, I had community service, joined a local rotary club, had a child. Plus, I had a car. I mean really, why run? I HAD A CAR.

Perhaps this was the natural outgrowth of aging from youthful ability: I AM fit, I CAN run. Why do I need to keep running?

As we all know, fitness doesn't last forever. Well, we know it when we hit forty. For those of you still under forty, you suck. Oh, and a bit of advice for when you get to that age: PREPARE FOR THY DOOM.

My spouse changed all that non-running nonsense(as they often do. I mean the change part, not the running part. The fact that she picked running is just 'lucky' I guess). She was motivated to lose weight and we started a self-induced Body-For-Life regimen, running for just 20 minutes three times a week. We were running about nine or ten minute miles back then. No big deal. I despised it, but I love her, so whadayado? Ah, courtship.

We followed that program, did weight training every other day, followed the accompanying diet, and lost weight. For eight weeks, we saw great results, and then she got pregnant, which of course ruined everything. I know that I was secretly happy to stop running, even if she was sad about it. Run? While pregnant? That's just crazy.

So another break, which lasted for years, really, until the last couple years when honey dragged my sorry butt outside again and we began shuffling our way to fitness.

And just what, pray tell, are these ludicrous ideas that so-called 'real' runners keep throwing around like they actually exist? Runner's High? Second Wind?

*Runner's high*? This is a cruel joke they tell newbies so they'll keep running. They fool us into thinking we must just not "get it". The runner's high seems like the emperor's new clothes to me, something only the smart can see. Clearly I am too stupid, and it just looks like a dude running up the street sucking wind. Naked.

*Second wind*? To me, that's like one of those political terms cooked up to make something sound better than it is, like death tax, or job creators. My second wind consists of a five minute period that I am not gasping desperately for breath. I think, suddenly, "Hey, I might not fall on my face immediately on the next step! I think this must be that second wind thing everyone talks about!" And then the feeling passes and I DO fall flat on my face. I believe runners call this "the wall", or as I call it "the living death."

Let's note here that second wind sounds like a bit of an oxymoron, like "military intelligence." The term implies you had a first wind. That there was wind at all. I guess I'm running to try to experience the second wind before I experience my "Last gasp."

As a kid, running was my happy place, but now it represents my grueling struggle against the forces of evil: fat. Gravity. Beer belly. Old age.

Running is the armor I wear to ward off these villains, but it is heavy. And it smells like old socks.

I hate running because it represents the sacrifices that characterize life as an adult: running is changing diapers. Running is doing the dishes, waking at 4:30am to catch a plane to get to that conference, washing the car, cleaning the garage. Running is work. Obligation. It is setting the burglar alarm. Yelling "get off my lawn!" Running, in short, represents every pain in the ass thing I have to do in my life. It is joyless.

Someday I will catch a glimpse of the glory of running again, relive a brief memory as a child, fleet of foot, carefree, running as fast as I could and totally aware of the wind flying past my face.

Wait. I almost had it there.

Ah.

Nope.


Until that time, I'll keep throwing one foot in front of the other in a vain attempt to better myself and ward off the forces of evil. (read: fatness)

No wonder old men get grumpy. They've run so much!

I had a thought. Why not try to see if I can jump-start my love of running? Defibrillate my old feelings for running through a forced experiment. Why not see if I can rekindle an old flame?

So I created a 30-day challenge for that purpose. What's more, I made a very rash decision to actually follow through with it.

Goodbye youthful running idiot. Hello old-age running idiot.

## The rules of my 30-day self-challenge:

- Thou must run every day. Thine runs must be 30 minutes. Even if thine heart says "no," and thine feet are reduced to bloodiness.
- Thou must wear your Sportswatch, but thou canst not look at it. On paine of death.
- Thou will record your activity results honestly, every day. Weight. Distance. Time.
- Thou must write your thoughts as they happen, or dictate those thoughts into a futuristic recording device to be put to pen later.
- Thou mayest walk if need be. Thou art not a robot, FFS.
- Thou must be optimistic. Thou must be OPTIMISTIC, DAMMIT!

## Why would you subject yourself to this?

Why indeed. As a self-proclaimed hater of running, why would I go through with this idiotic experiment?

Running 30 days in a row is a grand experiment, isn't it? Just a couple days before I started, I googled the idea. Of COURSE it's not original. Triathletes do it to build endurance.

I am not a triathlete. The idea of being in a triathlon is fantastic. Also, being shot in a cannon to Jupiter, also fantastic. Or waking up and finding out I am Captain Marvel. Fantastic. A triathlon is real enough, it's theoretically possible for it to happen, but then there's that whole swimming part. I have the swimming skills of a cat. With no legs. A dead cat with no legs.

So nope, uh nope, and nope.

I also have a bit of time on my hand. I'm a consultant, which is a fancy way of saying I'm not working right now, and am a "gun for hire" when needs be. I'm a business mercenary. I'm a 46 year old guy with an MBA, but right now there aren't a lot of business wars that need me. So why not try to improve myself while I have some time?

I don't consider myself a runner. My wife, now *she's* a runner. She completed 13 half-marathons in 2013. I ran a couple 5k's with her, and a 10k. She isn't competitive about it, but she runs several times a week. In fact, she's quite irritable if she doesn't. I run 1 or 2 times per week. "ish." Sometimes I go back to zero times a week just to remind myself what I am capable of. I think I have run as many as 4 times a week.

Never more. My average distance is probably right at three miles. My average pace is around an eleven minute mile. Yeah, I am not breaking any speed records, though when I want to turn it on I can get to around a 7 minute pace. For about 200 yards.

Most importantly, I wanted to answer some questions, and putting my body through hell seemed like a good way to answer them:

- Can I run for 30 days in a row? Is it possible? Or will I end at day eight with blisters and blood?
- Will I lose weight if I don't make significant changes in diet? This has been my hope for a long time.
- Can I begin to experience the runner's high? Will running help me get more "clarity" in my life?
- Can I start to love running again? Or, alternatively, will I be "cured" of running forever?
- 

It's November 1st, 2014. Here. We. Go.

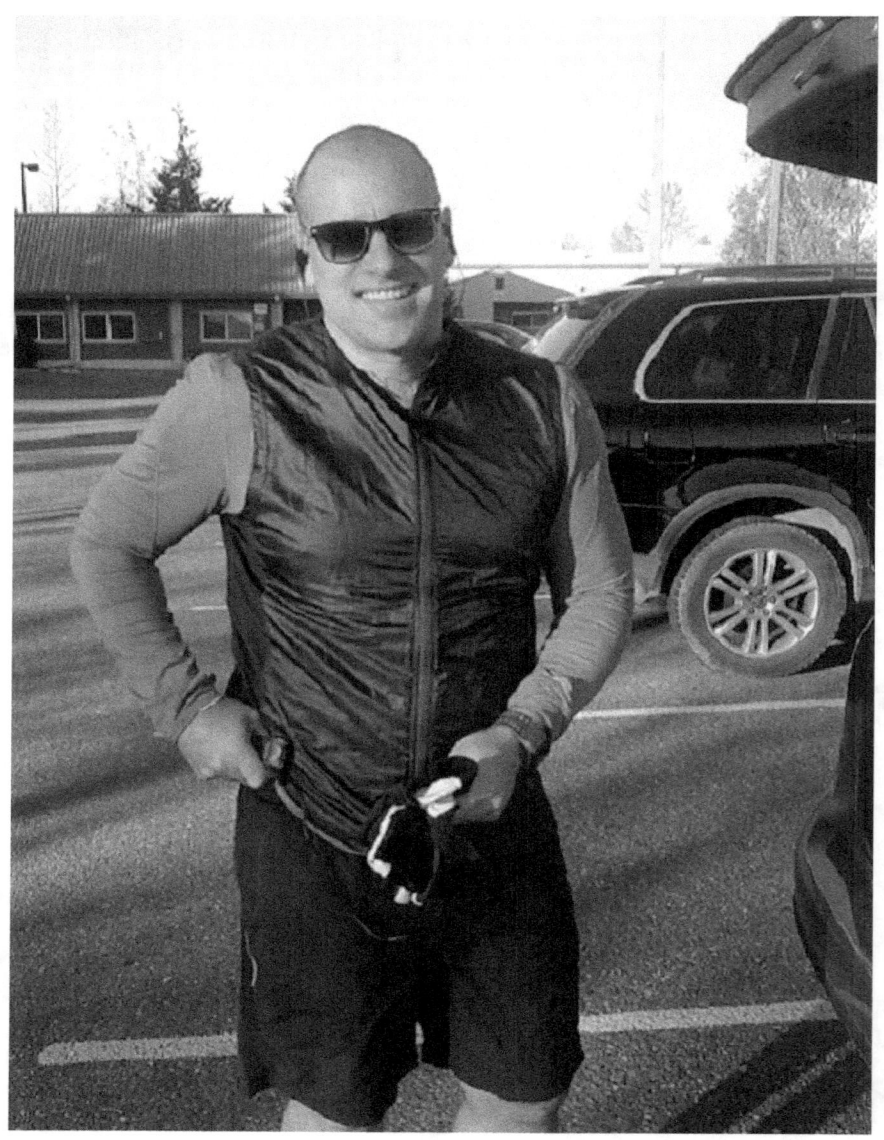

Tony in a Pre-sucking-wind moment.

# 1. "A QUESTION THAT SOMETIMES DRIVES ME HAZY: AM I OR ARE THE OTHERS CRAZY?" – ALBERT EINSTEIN

I weighed in at 241 pounds this morning – that's pretty close to an average weight for me over the last five years. It is the day after Halloween. I head out to Snohomish, Washington to a nature preserve. It looks to be about a three mile run on the Snohomish county parks' map. We live in Mukilteo, just north of Seattle, and Snohomish is about 15 minutes away towards the Cascade Mountains.

I'm nervous. You'd think if you planned on doing something for 30 days in a row, you wouldn't be nervous day one, but I've never tried this before – it's a pretty big step, so yeah, even running two miles today I'm pretty nervous for what the future holds.

It's foggy out today, kind of a high thick fog. A fine November day in the Pacific Northwest. My car says its 48 degrees Fahrenheit, which seems very chilly. I'm wearing shorts.

And I'm excited. Not because I'm wearing shorts. That would be weird. Actually, being excited and wearing shorts have nothing to do with each other. The fact that they were in proximity to each other was a bit of a mistake, actually. I regret that.

I am chasing something with this idea: a kind of mental clarity. My wife talks about this all the time (she's the real runner in the family). She talks about how running tends to be her happy place, and while I've also had those moments of lucidity, it's much rarer for me. So I'd like to continue to experience that as part of this exercise. In fact, part of the purpose of this exercise to see if running every day helps generate that automatically as part of a run. Scott Jurek, in his book Eat & Run, talks about ultra-marathoning and how that's definitely part of the chase for ultra-marathoners too, and how he can experience that runner's high four or five times in a race of that length. To Mr. Jurek I say "thanks but no thanks," but the question remains: will running every day help me get at least partially to this elusive running nirvana?

I'd also like to see if I feel that in my very thoughts, in dictating and in reviewing my dictation for this project, seem to become more coherent. That's in addition to all the other weight loss and fitness goals that are wrapped up in this whole thing, some of which are:

- Can I survive?
- Can I lose weight?
- Can I experience the runner's high?
- Can I become more conditioned for running?
  Finally,
- Can I find this stupid place I'm running today?

I'm a bit lost.

(Consulting phone)

Okay, I made it here. The Bob Hierman Wildlife Park at Thomas' Eddy. Well that's a mouthful. As you come into the park, there is a little motor home parked at the side for what must be the Park "Ranger." That's rather hilarious, actually, for a county park just outside the city limits and in a pretty swank residential area filled with horse paddocks and cow pasture.

If I were the ranger, I would be using that line all the time at bars. "I have a trailer at the 'wildlife preserve,' you know what I mean? I live where life is wild, baby." In my mind the ranger is not so subtle with the pickup lines. Also, I would use the term "Ranger" in a vaguely Army way, not in a "park" way. If you know what I mean, baby.

It's a cool clear day. I have my music. The fog is lifting. It's not raining. Looks to be a stunning landscape.

So I begin.

Whoops, ha, forgot to sync my nike+ sportswatch with the satellite. Okay, just a moment for that.

*Jeopardy music plays.* 5 minutes later.*

Okay, so I'm not using my sportswatch today since it can't seem to TomTom up with the Satellite. Haven't we figured this technology out yet? If the search for the Airline lost in Malaysia is an indicator, apparently, the answer is "no." But I'll just hit the stop watch and that will be fine.

Okay so NOW I begin…

Part of the idea here is to "experience" running again, not just slogging along as some difficult thing I have to do because I'm old and fat(guilty!), but to experience it as something that's joyful, something that allows me to get out and commune with nature. So I try to look around more as I come down the hill, passing a small lake. I look in the distance at a low tree that looks to be the perfect habitat for eagles, though I don't see any eagles or a nest. It's a marshy field to either side of the path for the first one-third of a mile to the river, then the path bends left and runs along the bank.

But then the trail changes. It's the first day and I have apparently picked the muddiest trail I have ever been on. This wilderness trail features a lot of wilderness. Very little trail. I duck overgrown branches, hanging blackberries, and run along the sides of the trail dodging mud patches. It does remind me, however, that running is a primal feature of being an animal. We run to get to things, or to get away from things.

So the next question is: am I running TO something when I run, or am I running away from something?

Well, my podrunner music rocks me along to the halfway point. Which is a fishing area, a gravel spit along the Snohomish River. The river is very high, but there's no fisherman. Just me, though I saw an older couple that might be a bit lost, asking me if this is a loop. I told them it is an out-and-back. But you could get a bit lost in there. I've been mentally marking the landmarks to turn back along. I can't believe what the guide says was listed as one and a half miles out, but I've only dodged and weaved for twelve minutes to this point.

So I take another little trail to try to extend my run around the spit. It ends immediately. Fantastic.

You know, clarity is very important to someone who wants to write something. In conversation we tend to be all over the place even in the middle of a sentence. We might have other conflicting, branching, parallel thoughts we could "go down," but as we speak, or as we write(especially as we write since speech tends to be more forgiving), we have to stay on the same track and pull that thought through to its end, to a conclusion, or just to the next sentence. But that's hard to do without focus.

I ran into that "lost" couple as they doubled back to the river. I jokingly asked them if they were lost yet, but they seem fine. That is, she seemed fine, but the man seemed absolutely wasted. Drunk. Hey, if you're going to get out on a walk on Saturday morning, why make it a LOT more fun, right?

I'm beginning my muddy ascent back. This is a dangerous muddy trail. I keep thinking about how I rarely lose my balance, but I don't want to think about that too much or I'll definitely end up on my butt somewhere in the mud.

So here's a question: if as a runner, you're looking for clarity, is it better to run on a smooth surface, a trail, with people or without them? FreeRunning is a whole movement, right?

By the way, there's a reason that not very many good Free Runners come out of the Pacific Northwest. Vaulting over a stump is very impressive, but catapulting into the patch of blackberries on the other side has probably made a PNW Free runner or two consider the wisdom of launching themselves through obstacles. Ouch.

I have a theory on that last idea: how to "induce" that clear moment, and whether a trail or flat surface would be better. It's based on some of what Method acting teaches actors. An actor tries to experience something "real", but it isn't real. An acting exercise I always enjoyed was to count pennies while you recite your lines. By "distracting" yourself from your own hang-ups and inhibitions, you can generate a bit of neutrality emotionally, which helps you to experience things differently. That's a fancy way of saying I think trails would be better. Trails make you focus a tiny bit. A piece of your mind has to concentrate on how your feet are hitting the trail, which might help to get you into that yogi-like zen state, which could help induce a bit of the runner's high. That's a day one observation for ya. Absolutely no clinical evidence to back that up whatsoever. Call it a theory. Let's see if any part of that plays out over the next 29 days, or whether if I'm full of hooey.

I've had these shoes for a couple months. This is by far the dirtiest I've ever gotten them. What was once a bright orange is now stained brown with mud.

Isn't it funny how you can do things without resolve, just for fun, and everything's fine? At that moment you make a resolution, though, something changes, once you put your head down, all of a sudden it's the most difficult thing you've ever done. There's a psychology behind that, I'm sure. I think it has to do with inertia.

Here we go. It's an idyllic run, downhill to the Snohomish river front. That is, idyllic until the return: a grueling climb up the same hill. I hate out-and-backs.

I'm back, gasping for breath. Total Time On Feet(TOF) 24 minutes ten seconds. Probably about two miles, but I wouldn't be surprised if it was a bit farther. I have to go home and mapquest this thing to see how far it was. It's my first run, I'm counting it, dangit, I went to the end of the trail and back. Accomplishment Number one!

Clarity? Not really. We'll see if I can kinda get in the zone, but my thoughts weren't anything too spectacular, now were they? If I really get in the zone, I'll cure Cancer. That's how this works, right?

I drive home to meet my wife, who has completed her seven mile run on the Burke-Gilman trail in Seattle. Showoff. She asks me how my run was? Good, I said, muddy little trail, but I did 24 minutes. "24 minutes?" She asks. Yeah, probably about two miles. "Well," she says "you only have six minutes to go." Haha. Uh, what? "I thought you were going to do 30 minutes of running?"

Crap.

So I put down my cup of coffee fresh from the microwave, put my muddy shoes back on, and head outside to our neighborhood. What an idiot. I forgot my own stupid rule day ONE. Chucklehead.

There's nothing more laborious in life than going back to finish off a task you thought was completed. I owed finishing this run to myself – and of course I owed it to my adoring public, thank you so much! – and I run for a whopping six more minutes so I can say I actually did it. I suppose that technically I could go on two fifteen-minute runs every day, but who the heck wants to do that? So <u>NOW</u> the run is done and I can go have date night with my wife, have a delicious beer or two and get ready for day two.

**Day 1 Results:**
    Weight: 241
    Total distance: 2.2 miles
    Total TOF: 30 minutes
    Weather/terrain: brisk and muddy
    Attitude: Just fine thanks. Okay, a bit crappy. Well, you asked.

## Competitive Spirit

When I ~~won the Western States Ultramarathon~~ placed 811th in the 2nd annual Totetum Shore 5k Fun walk/run, I had a sudden realization.

I might never win a race.

Like, *EVER*.

I am competitive by nature, and I find my self-talk during a run is often focused on doing more and better. Comedian Jim Gaffigan talks about it too: "when I'm working out I tell myself I'm going to do this every day. Then the next day I'm like 'well, not EVERY day.' Then the next day I'm like… 'I'm happy with the way I look.'"

I watch my time, thinking about how I can run farther, faster, better. But I'm getting older, you know? Being competitive seems rather far-fetched. I am no longer at that place in my life, but my brain latches on to it, like it's the only reason to run. It's not.

## 2. "THE HEART HAS ITS REASONS, BUT THE MIND MAKES THE EXCUSES." - AMIT ABRAHAM

All Right, it's November second, we just finished watching the New York Marathon, so I'm going to try to use that for inspiration.

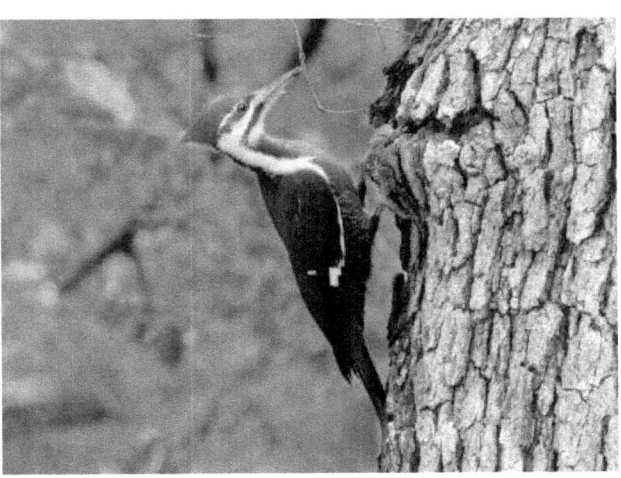

As I head outside there is a pileated woodpecker going to town on a tree next to our house. It's a cool day, overcast but no fog. No rain but cooler by a bit than yesterday's 48 degrees.

I'm going to run "Big Gulch" today, a picturesque 3 mile trail run that starts at our house. It's really wonderful to have a trail run accessible so close, no driving necessary. We'll see if we can get my watch to sync up today.

Only slight soreness today, and I'm listening to "TranceContinental" on my iPod, a dance mix at 170 BPM. "oontz, oontz, oontz"

This run starts out with an undulating sidewalk run, uphill and downhill for the first mile. Mostly downhill, with only a couple blocks of climbing. After that, a quick 200' ascent on a trail through a community park makes it good trail-running fun.

I was ambivalent about watching the marathon this morning. As inspiring as it is to watch these people run 26 miles, they do it by running at a five to six-minute pace the ENTIRE race. I couldn't run a five minute mile to save my life. They're bounding along as if they are practically walking at that clip. A bear chasing me couldn't get me going that fast. If you tied ten thousand dollars to the front of a car and said I could have it if I ran behind it and grabbed it clean, which would take a five minute mile, that money is safe. If you tied someone on the train tracks, and in order to save them I would have to get to them with a five minute mile, okay, well, you get the idea. It's not happening. The marathoners in the NYC marathon were inspiring, but the whole thing was a little daunting as well.

I really like this run because in the first mile the vistas are incredible as you wend down into a neighborhood near the water. 180 degree views of Puget Sound greet you, with the water line a hundred feet below you, and whether it's pouring rain or pouring sun, it's always an incredible sight. Today it's pouring sun

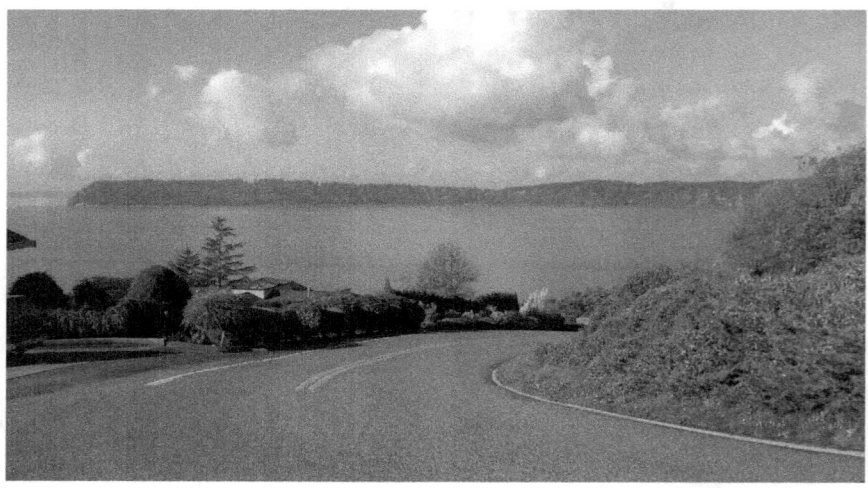

The thing I have to work really hard at is *slowing down*. I was fast as a kid, but in the interim between youth and middle age, I lost all the ability to run fast, but not the mentality behind it. So as a runner(or as someone who might someday become one) I really try to discipline

myself to NOT go all out from the start of the run, to try to set a sustainable pace up front.

You don't think about that as a kid. You don't think "how long can I maintain this pace?"

You just want to run.

So it's an evolution of patience. Running a marathon is favorable to people who are older because they have the patience to train for it. It's a change from the desire for instant gratification that motivates us in our youth to a more patient approach to life, and to running. Suddenly it's not about finishing first, it's about finishing at all. In this way the running journey is also a recognition of our mortality. Because none of us are going to get out of all this alive. And for the record, I am not so keen on finishing "first" in life, if you know what I mean.

I'm almost to the bottom of the first hill, and I'm thinking about something else I am gunning for; a 23-mile hike through the woods next summer. Hopefully, I'll be in shape enough to run most of it and finish it in one day. It's a climb through cascade pass. By all reports, one of the most spectacular views in Washington, and that's saying something. We have lots of 'em.

Now the hill. I've only made it up this hill a couple times without stopping. In fact, for a while when we moved here last year, I just made it to the base of the hill before I had to stop. It gassed me that much, often still does. Now I know I have the capability, and quitting is a little bit optional for me.

This 200 foot incline is broken up into three distinct pieces of switchback. I make it up two of them today. Actually, as I reflect on it, I did okay and then I saw a man walking his Labrador. They stopped on the side of the road as his well-trained dog just sat next to the trail. That was nice. Somewhere in my brain I decided it was okay to stop. Isn't it funny how sometimes any excuse is excuse enough to get you to back off from the goal you've set for yourself? Any excuse will work:

A man walks across the street to his neighbor's house and asks "can I borrow your axe?"

"No," says his neighbor. "I'm making soup."

"Making soup? What does that have to do with borrowing your axe?"

"Nothing. But I don't want to lend you my axe, so what difference does it make what excuse I use?"

We all have excuses for things we don't want to do. "I don't have time", "I can't run that far"

Today, the hill got me. It usually does. I made soup. Whatever. Don't judge.

For my goal, again I have to remind myself that my goal is running for 30 days. Not setting a new personal record(PR) every day in terms of pace or running as far as I can. I'm only trying to set one record: consistency.

Top of the first big hill now. It angles down for another one-third mile until a slow climb begins, punctuated with a big gnarly set of stairs at the end. I should count the stairs today.

Over the last year and a half, this run is the one I've done most frequently, so there are no surprises here. There are plenty of hills, however. The Pacific Northwest is a great place to learn to run hills. As I mentioned yesterday, it's not so great a place to free run through the woods. In Big Gulch, there's a lovely little bottom part of the trail where the Mukilteo sewer line comes out, so there's a lovely pocket of methane there. There aren't enough fans in the world to blow that smell out. It's always pervasive. As General Patton said: "When in Hell, keep going." So this low spot is never where you want to stop.

I run through it, breathing through my mouth.

After college I spent a lot of time reading the great thinkers in the Positive Thinking movement. Norman Vincent Peale. Napoleon Hill. Orison Swet Marden. A lot of my base of understanding life, my ideological core, believes the idea that if you work hard enough, keep your goals before you, then you have a better possibility of achieving them. That has been sorely tested over the last ten months of doing more business consulting. Sometimes find myself in a bit of a tailspin, mentally. Failure definitely tests you in unexpected ways. That is part of the reason I'm setting this goal before me, to continue to apply myself, to structure my approach to something and go after it with commitment.

There are no commitments like the ones you make to yourself. And none more important – or more difficult – to keep.

I stop to give a talk to three people with three dogs walking off-leash. Actually, I amiably say "I'm okay with this but if my wife were here she would be freaking out right now." That is absolutely true. They respond with "if it didn't seem okay, we would put them on-leash." But how do you know, dog owners? How do you know if someone is afraid of dogs? Do they have to cringe and pull back in fear for you to understand it? That, incidentally, is one of the main reasons that my wife doesn't run trail runs by herself. That and the oppressively scary prospect of some maniac jumping out of the bushes at her. She's afraid of dogs and maniacs. Also maniac dogs. She doesn't want any part of them.

The moral of the story is that it's all well and good to let your dogs off-leash, but if you're terrorizing other people with it, then you might want to re-think your strategy. There are all kinds of stories in the news – of course MY dogs would never do this, and neither would yours –

stories of dogs attacking, maiming, and even killing runners. Maybe we should keep ours on a leash, right?

This is reminiscent of my son, who has a peanut allergy. That was discovered when he ate a peanut butter cracker in day care. He blew up like a balloon and had to be rushed to the hospital. A lot of parents are pretty upset about rules regarding allergies in the classroom, and they don't think it should affect them or their kids. We are fortunate in that our son doesn't have an "inhaled" allergy, it's just ingestion in his case. Again, the point is that if your son's lunch is a threat to my son's life, I would respectfully ask that you pack a different lunch. So with our canine friends. Leashing is an appreciated courtesy to other humans.

I think sometimes I know that I'm feeling the runner's high because I feel like I can run some more. How would I know that except for the fact that you had already stopped for a walk break, right? So of course I take walk breaks, because if you don't take walk breaks, you can't have a runner's high. Seems legit.

My wife disagrees with me, by the way. Act surprised. I talked to her this morning about my challenge, and she reminded me that two years ago, she set a challenge for herself to run five miles a day for a month. Of course she nailed it. She didn't lose weight. That's discouraging. Five miles. So of course my goal seems paltry in comparison.

She disagrees with me on the trail running vs. road running and clarity. She would rather run on a flat surface to get in the zone. It's a good thing I'm smarter and have more degrees than her or I would be threatened by her superior intellect. Smarty-pants.

Here's the stairs.

86 stairs.

Did you run up them Tony?

Heck no.

From the park at the top of the stairs, it's a half-mile of sidewalk back to the house, with a slight uphill and downhill. Running this part is usually pretty easy – it's that last bit before you finish, and the "joy" of being done carries me through. Go ahead and use air quotes around "joy" right now. Now you feel my sarcasm.

Finished! I had a good run, sarcasm or no. Definitely felt some of the runner's high today and enjoyed myself after the bridge at mile two, just before the stairs. I did have to focus a lot on the stairs. In retrospect, it seems that my dictation starts slow and then gains speed and focus as I run. I also have more interesting thoughts to share in general.

## Day 2 Results
Weight: 243
Miles: 2.91
Average Pace: 12. per mile
TOF: 37.09 minutes
"Way to get out there!" Says my watch, in an attempt to be inspirational. It says I burned 528 calories too, so that's like burning off one Halloween candy. Wait, stay positive. I did it! Day two in the books!

## Quitting is Optional

By the way, I do feel that quitting is always optional, but I always have "walk breaks" when I run. Right now I can only run about two miles on a pretty level surface before I feel like I have to stop. I tried to think of the truth: that quitting is optional. Let's face it, unless you're falling to the ground, you can still run slowly. Unless your legs are absolutely giving way, and you're face-planting, you can move a little more slowly at a sustained running pace. Quitting is optional, because if it isn't optional, you're probably having some kind of cardiac event.

With that said, it's an option you might want to take. I mean, I'm running for health, not to become a competitive heptathlete. I'm a person not a danged robot. I'm running for fun, not to make myself miserable. So if I want a break, well consarned it, I'm takin' one.

## 3. "IF YOU WANT TO GO RUNNING WITH ME, YOU SHOULD BE PREPARED TO WALK A LOT."

Pouring. Huzzah.

If you live in the Pacific Northwest, especially western Washington and Oregon, rain isn't exactly newsworthy. It's still depressing, at times. You have to try and embrace it, because it's not going away anytime soon.

So of course I picked the month of November, the wettest month of the year. Well done, Tony. *golf clap*

My bad.

Regardless of the rain, and in spite of it, I start my run at Eleven a.m. today, upbeat and energetic about running. That's a little weird.

It's day three, it is a wet, wet day – wet enough that I'm actually wearing a rain slicker to run in. That's really par for the course, a normal NW drippy day. I'm running from a starting point in McCollum Park, which follows a bike path right through the city of Mill Creek, Washington. It's the run my wife and I used to do with friends before we moved from Everett, so it's very familiar. My watch is actually synced up with the satellite, so that looks like it's going to work, I'm going to make a little loop around the park and take off and meet a friend for lunch in Mill Creek.

I thought day 3 was about the time I'd be all "GOD, THIS IS A PAIN IN MY BUTT," but I seem to have a pretty good attitude about it. Looking forward to my third day and seeing if I can maintain it, mostly. Which is another strange thing, this excitement I have for being consistent about this.

So here we go!

It's funny listening to my dictations again, as I gasp and pant for breath. Sounds like I'm going to keel over. But I have high hopes today, since this is a rather flat run, I should be able to run most of this thing without a problem, even in my advancing age and decrepitude. Quitting is optional, right? *gasp*

I'm splashing through mud puddles on the perimeter of the park, running through a brilliant green and crimson canopy of the trees.

It's impossible (as I wend my way up a small hill) to talk about weight loss and exercise without talking about diet in the discussion. And I want to talk about my diet. Not because I'm proud of it, but because it sucks. I have a long-standing theory if I focus solely on exercise, I can make up for any deficiencies in my diet. A part of me knows this is bullcrap. As the saying goes: "you can't outrun a beer." I do like beer.

I want to talk about my diet because sometimes when I am running it seems that I can feel the toxins and the impurities burning off me. That's just how I perceive the delightful sweat/BO smell that accompanies my runs. It might be better, I recognize, if I didn't put those toxins into my body in the first place?

I don't smoke. I used to(I was a theater major, it was part of the curriculum), but then I went and got married, and my wife is smarter than that.

I'm getting a recurring theme in the first three days, aren't you? "My wife is awesome and I'm a bit of a slug." Ha ha. A good marriage is about two people drawing out the best in each other, and I'd like to think that I draw out the best in her, just as she draws out the best in me. Or is this is a convenient fiction we have created to make us feel better? Whatever, its love so shut up.

I don't normally run with a rain slicker, but this one is great. This is a slicker that captures a bit of heat and reflects it back, it's light and comfortable. Running in the cold and rain is a bit of a balancing act as you try to find that balance between overheating and getting too cold. I'm not a proud man(well, not too proud?), and I have run many times with a plastic bag on. I usually sandwich it between layers, so I rustle when I walk but can still look the fashion plate that I am. A thirteen gallon kitchen bag with a few holes in it makes a dry shirt between layers; I'd just rip it off at the appropriate time when I get too warm and don't have too much farther to go. My family doesn't really go for this plan – I think its ego. Even with the kids. They think it's a silly idea. It's man versus nature out here, and I'm not too proud to say that I'd rather be more comfortable than less comfortable, and nature is more powerful than I am.

I'm at a turn on the path at one mile, winding next to a Native Growth Protection Area(NGPA) behind upscale apartments. The path is slippery with leaves; it could be a function of my footfall and running mechanics that I never seem to slip on them. Or the fact that I am slow as heck. You can't slip if you aren't moving.

## Into the Wild

There was a book that came out some years ago: "Into the Wild," about a young man named Chris McCandless(I think of "McCandless" as I run through McCollum park!). The story of Chris McCandless became popular lore when an article ran on him in Outside magazine. He was a somewhat misunderstood, loner-type character, personable, but so taken with the outdoors that he had a dream of living alone in the wilderness. The dream of a frontiersman. I grew up in Alaska, so I can absolutely relate to his desires. The article sparked two different sentiments for most people: one was "oh what a fool", and the other was "he was a poor misguided boy, why would he do that?"
Growing up in Alaska, I have to say I fall into the former camp: I considered it rather stupid.
Since then, the author John Krakauer has a bestselling book and a movie about the Chris McCandless story, and has discovered more recently that McCandless might have fallen prey to a specific type of neurotoxin. Krakauer doesn't hold hope that this discovery will change the way most Alaskan's feel about McCandless, and he's right. McCandless wasn't dumb because he failed to recognize a neurotoxin. He was dumb because he challenged nature on her home turf and paid the price for it.
From Krakauer's recounting of his life, Chris McCandless seemed like a smart kid. But Nature will eat you up and spit you back out. I understood his dream, but it's not a good idea to go off half-cocked into Mother Nature as McCandless did. In Alaska you can wander off in the woods to go to the bathroom and stumble through the ice on a small creek, and suddenly you are in a life-or-death situation. It's very unforgiving, peeing in Alaska.
As I have always said, "it's all fun and games until someone ingests a bunch of neurotoxin. "
Too soon? The point is that McCandless challenged nature. You work with nature, not against it. I try to remind myself of that as I work to better myself through this experiment. Sometimes it's hard to remember that this isn't man versus nature every second of the run. It's man versus himself.
My run becomes more difficult. One foot in front of another. The journey of a thousand miles begins with a single step. Here comes the downhill just before mile two, a rough run so far, but I have that sense of

accomplishment that comes from doing what I hate.

I'm meeting a friend of mine for lunch. He helps train police officers. We set this loose timeline around lunch, but I'm not worried about it. He was in the military, he went to Iraq, so I know that despite the fact that I left my car a few miles back he'll be there.

Moments of clarity came early this run. Now it's a slog. When it's a struggle like this, I want to look at my watch. That can be a precursor to stopping, but I'm not letting myself do it. I've run this before, and I know the run. Pace doesn't matter. Time doesn't matter, except that I am running for 30 minutes, and I know it's not close to 30 minutes. So why should I look?

My pre-run diet this morning before I began running around 11:00 was four cups of coffee, a banana, and an apple. Not the best preparation. Talking about it leads me to a bit of a bonk(can you bonk fifteen minutes in?), but I'm going to keep running, dangit.

Okay, stopping. That was twenty minutes of a good pace, but suddenly I want to crawl into bed with my teddy bear.

This run was unlike the first couple of runs in that I felt pretty clear of mind early on. As I hit a twenty minute "bump" and have to take a walk break, however, I am feeling pretty wiped out.

Isn't it funny how we have to eat all the time? You can't skip meals or it really affects you. It's very difficult to fast. One of the few things I know about my estranged Dad is that he used to experiment with this kind of weirdness: water and food consumption. That's an interesting thing to challenge yourself with if you don't have to, isn't it? Diet for no reason? He would go without food for a period of time. Reportedly, according to my Mom, he said that going without food was tough, but going without water was much tougher. I should note that I don't believe my dad had weight issues of any kind. He just wanted to challenge himself.

I'm thinking about Teriyaki or a Gyro. An illusory smell of teriyaki in my nostrils will surely propel me for the last half mile.

It's about a two-minute walk break. Walk breaks are such an interesting thing. I think we all know people that seem to be able to sit at a desk all day and then suddenly they think they should exercise and they turn into these fat supermen that can run for eight miles. Just on a whim.

I laugh about that – I'm not going to "accidentally" run eight miles. Ever. On a whim? That's not an accident, it's a danged commitment. The idea of running that far regularly is daunting, almost unimaginable. Is this my excusitis acting up? *cough* I think I have excusitis.

And by the way, for those of you who say you can't run two miles, or are the person who says "there's no way I can get there," just get on your feet. Just walk it. Of COURSE it doesn't burn as *many* calories, but it does burn calories. It will help make you more fit. If you have problems with all your friends that are so dang fast or run so often, and you're old and fat, just get there and be old and fat on your feet for as many miles as you can. It's your fitness, not theirs. You set the bar, and whether or not you achieve it is up to you, your body and mind.

Okay, pep talk over.

I see a blue heron skipping across the lake as I finish my run with a long walk. I am totally wiped, but I'm still upright. I'm feeling a little rubbery-legged. Was it that I didn't eat enough? Or it could be I'm not ready for this every day commitment. I will keep up with it. I mean come on, 30 minutes. It can't be this hard every day. I'm still a bit out of breath just walking. I shake my head in disbelief at my lack of conditioning. It's not a marathon for pete's sakes.

It's a gristle and bone kind of run on day three. Started off well, but I struggled. Gut check.

I meet my friend for a bento box and talk about his work. I try not to mention how weakass I am.

I top a crappy run off later that evening by taking my kids to the soccer field and shooting goals, running drills with them. I anticipate that my soreness will get worse, but I take a hot bath to try and soak it away.

## Day 3 Results

Weight: 242
Miles: 2.47
TOF: 30 minutes 40 seconds
12:28 average pace

# 4. "WISELY AND SLOW. THEY STUMBLE THAT RUN FAST" – SHAKESPEARE

I have a friend that has done some landscaping work for us over the last couple of years. He's a friend because I met him as he worked on our yard and we hit it off. He's an old Pacific Northwest codger with a great sense of humor, loves hiking and being in the mountains, and can work like a donkey. Every so often he'll drop in at our house if he's working a landscaping job nearby. He stopped by today with an offer I can't refuse: a whole lot of flagstone from a place nearby… for free.

Awesome!

Now here's the bad news. Of course since it's free I have to help him unload it. That means day four starts out with a whole lot of working out for some free stuff and THEN I am going to go for my run/walk/drag myself by my bloody elbows. I'm a little sore from my ambitious attempt at playing soccer last night with a bit of cramping as I slept. This will be a true test, then.

More great news. I am up to 244 pounds, which means I am actually gaining weight so far. I don't really play the "watch the scale" game, but that's not an encouraging number either. At least I'm not wasting away to nothing.

Between unloading two loads of flagstone from the bed of Mark's pickup and a job interview call with a recruiter, its 1:00pm before I am able to hit the road on my already muddy legs. Another rainy day. Another barrel of laughs.

STAYING POSITIVE *forcing smile*

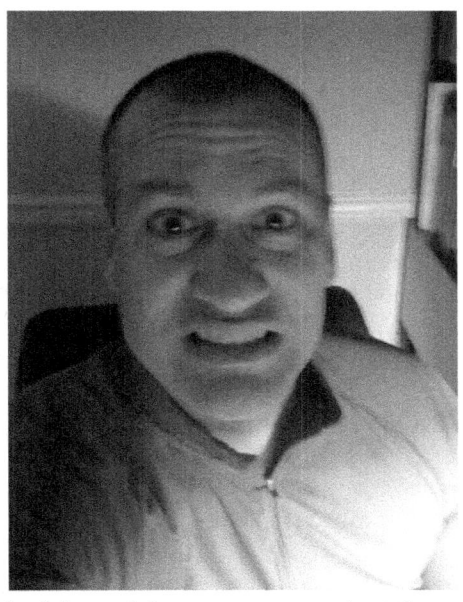

Oh yeah, that's very encouraging. That selfie isn't creepy at ALL.

Japanese gulch is a fantastic park in Mukilteo, about 800 acres with a railroad track running up one side. It's crisscrossed with trails up the side of the gulch and it's fairly easy to get lost in, unlike my normal run at Big Gulch with its two or three trailheads. It is bounded by residence at the top of the hill, a busy arterial at the entrance, and the Boeing Company property. The back end of the gulch presses up against the runway lights at the end of Paine Field. A little parking area and a small dog run are really the only features of the park besides the many loopy trails.

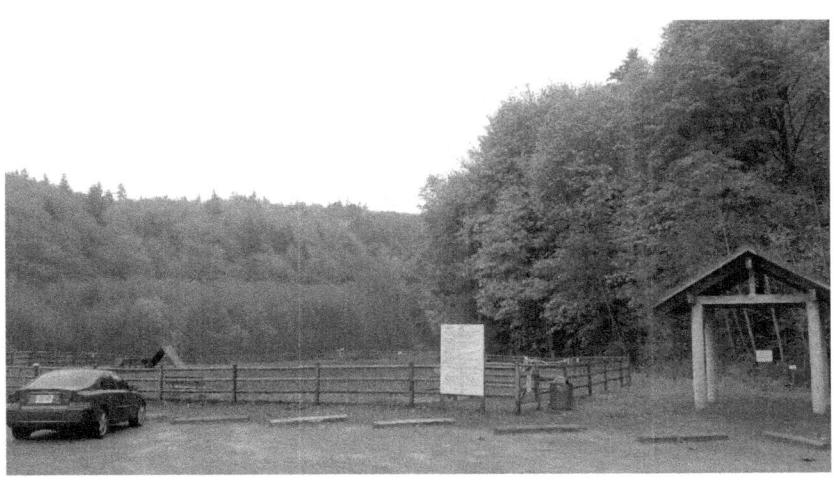

I'm going to try to take it easy on myself today and just go up and down the railroad tracks for the run. It will be a full run in terms of time on my feet, but I don't feel like slipping up and down the slopes in the mud. Japanese gulch features many trails which are little more than mud washouts, and they are so smooth with mud you can practically luge down them. If you're on foot, you might find yourself sliding down them on your rump. The trail starts off to the right, and I know it connects back across the stream to the railroad, so I start that way. It's an uphill grade on the way up, but coming back will feel like flying. I hope.

I have to confess at this point, I'm not very excited about this experiment. I'm definitely not feeling how "amazing" running is. I'm feeling how amazing it would be to stop. But hey, I'm giving it the time of day here. I'm not brushing running off because I have a prior commitment to clean my washing machine or floss my cat. I'm giving it the 30 days, because I'm wondering if being consistent will help me to fall in love with running again. So far, I've had flashes of brilliance, moments of clarity, but really I want to find out if the act of running over and over again helps me to do what my wife has done – to make running my own "happy place." Right now, it's not my happy place. It's my "oh my god I have to do this again" place.

I say all that and we're *only* on day four. This better not be 30 days of whining about running.

No pain, no gain? I like Jerry Seinfeld's response: "no pain, no pain."

As we all try to do things, early on the journey sucks. In another 26 days? It will be the most amazing thing I have ever done in my life. But right now, blech, blah, and bluh.

I'm heartened by one thing, however. There are so many books written by runners about running. What about the non-runner who wants to run? There are so many people who want to tell you how to improve your eight minute mile to a sub-six minute mile. People who want to recount their story about how they won the 2008 Monster Energy Drink Beijing marathon, or finished first in the Lucky Strike Iron Man.

What about us slow-as-slothy folks? Folks who can only run a few hundred yards at a time? There are no resources for this. Where are the books written by slow people FOR slow people? I'm encouraged that even if I come out of this experience with nothing more than a body that has aged a month more, I will have accomplished something by sticking to a goal. I will have proven that even a slow-ass non-runner like moi can get going.

We're not competitive runners. We are weaksauce. And we are proud.

Oprah Winfrey runs eight minute miles. I mean COME ON.

I start running, winding up the trail, hugging the right slope of the gulch.

I quickly realize that I have underestimated the slope on this side of the trail. It doesn't present as a gentle slope up to a field filled with butterflies, but rather an ass-kicking climb up Sadist hill.

I am 60 feet up the trail and still climbing when I pass a couple walking with their enormous Doberman off-leash. Thankfully, there is a fork in the trail back left and down here, so I say hello cheerfully and start down.

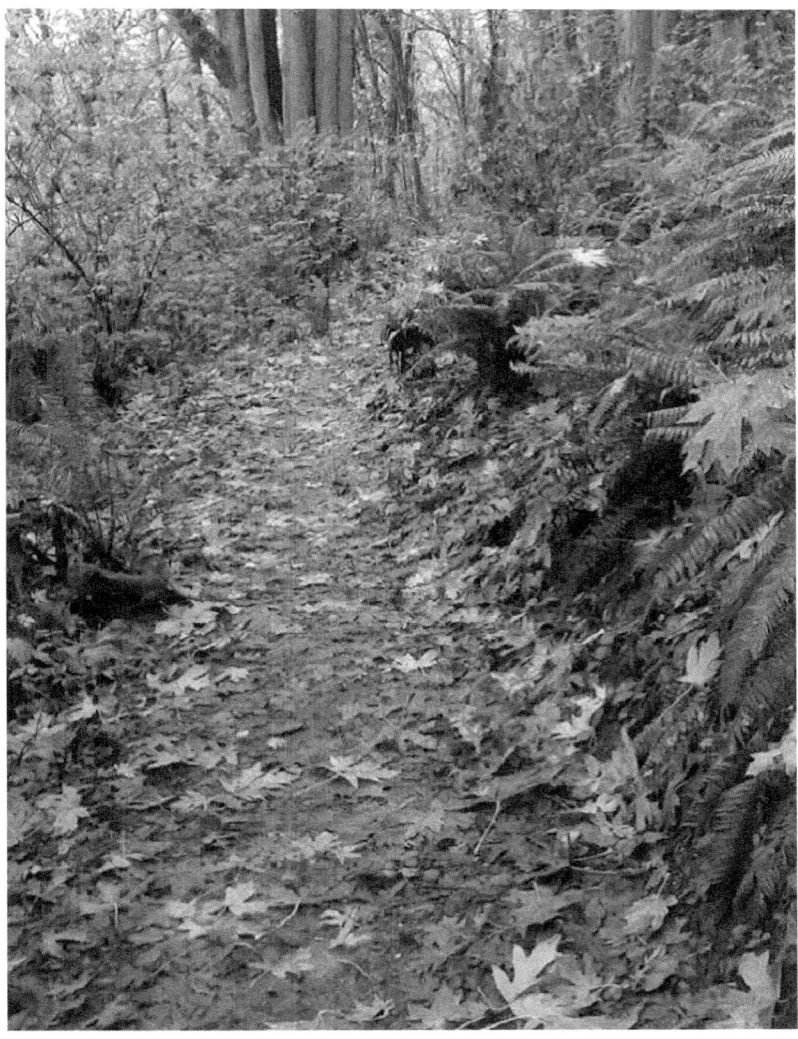

What I don't see is that the Doberman, who was another 30 feet on the other side of the fork, has started running towards me.

I hear them calling the dog and know he must be heading for me. I am carefully picking my way down a very muddy slope when I look back in time to see him leap past me towards a small bridge over a muddy spot.

He misjudges it. This large Doberman(who might only be couple years old) leaps off the mud towards the bridge, scaring the heck out of me in the process, but he gets the worst of the encounter. The mud sinks and he tumbles into and then onto the small wooden structure. He quickly rights himself, and runs back as quickly as he came. A flurry of mud and he's gone. "Good God," I mutter in stunned silence.

People. Do we have to have the "off leash" conversation again?

But I'm down off Doberman-friendly Sadist hill, Now I'm crossing the stream, which is very swollen, but at least back on a normal trail.

I definitely misjudged the elevation in general. I'm struggling and barely 10 minutes in. Forget about it. Focus.

I feel like I'm fighting for my life sometimes, running. That is probably not conducive to any kind of mental insight. Kicking in with the fight or flight response, that's not optimal. I need to slow down to get into more of a zone. I was just battling those hills. If you're trying to have fun running, uphill is not a good idea.

One of the neat things about living in Mukilteo is being so close to Boeing. Japanese Gulch is a great place to see some interesting planes taking off and landing, like the green one that flew overhead with a big "S7" on the tail. What I mistook for Chinese characters on the side were people:

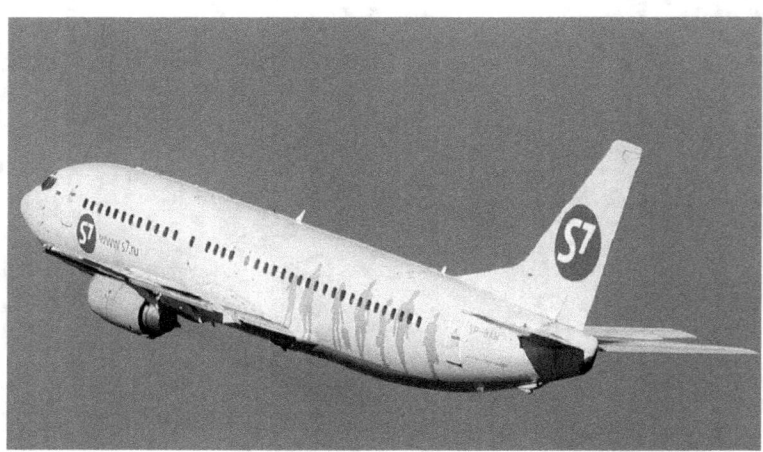

I'm running uphill next to a culvert placed there for water drainage, next to the tracks. I'm trying to keep my spirits up as I finish this ~~triathlon~~ short run. I don't know whose idea it was to run with these lead weights attached to my shoes, but it's definitely not helping.

Running up the railroad tracks reminds me of the story of "The Little Engine That Could", and it makes me wonder if it's possible to gain focus in yourself by repeating a mantra over and over. I'll have to try that sometime. Like "I think I can, I think I can."

Eighteen minutes in, I've taken a couple breaks, but I am feeling a bit stronger than I was on the hill. There is a gate here to go into Boeing property and the end of the runway markers. I may or may not finish my turnaround on private property. I can neither confirm nor deny it. That, dear reader, gives you "plausible deniability." In case anyone asks.

Turn-around time is at the 20 minute mark, and the rest is downhill, which means I should nail my negative split. That's a fancy runner way of saying that I can run the second half faster than the first.

Another writing and social media project I've been working on for a couple years is called "Dumberica,us" as in Dumb America. It's November 4th, Election Day today. There's an awful lot of comic material to work with on Election Day. Instead, I was thinking of Christmas in November. It's amazing to see all the store displays changing right after Halloween to Christmas decorations. Like, November first all the Halloween stuff is gone and it's time to buy Christmas lighting. Forget about Thanksgiving, we don't even do that anymore. Thanksgiving is getting the short end of the stick. There might be a few seasonal placemats out with cornucopias and fall fruit on them. Or a leftover pumpkin from Halloween, a last vestige. On Dasher, on Prancer! Push on with Christmas! Why? Well, Home Depot has to have stuff to sell displayed prominently, and Thanksgiving is a loser from a marketing perspective. I blame the mascot. Thanksgiving has weak promotional support.

I'm seeing the same plane twice, making another pass. Either that or it's Groundhog Day?

Running downhill is so great. It's practically effortless. It's like running on a treadmill, the ground moves itself. All you have to do is pick up your feet and let your body move.

Running downhill is like eating eggplant. No one likes eggplant, but if you put it in the right sauce, it's awesome. I don't like running, but you point me downhill and it doesn't *taste* like running, I like it, just as I like eggplant as long as it doesn't taste too much like eggplant.

I'm dying to look at my watch, but I dare not! It's like Sodom and Gomorrah. If I look at my watch, I'll turn into a pillar of salt. And stop.

I'm ready to keep it going with a little more running! Keep that negative split strong. I'm past my minimum at 32 minutes, but I'm not back to the park, so I keep going. Why not?

I finish my run with thoughts of the things that are important in my life: my family, my house. I find my mind wandering to work and career successes and failures, and the importance of those things seems very minor compared to the other things in my life I hold dear.

I find myself thinking of the opulence we have in our society, and that we shouldn't have homeless people any more. We have enough "things" in our society for everyone's basic needs. Heck, we have six homes sitting empty for each and every homeless person in America. John Naisbitt forecasted a housing glut in his book from 30 years ago, Megatrends. And they're using tires in third world countries to make homes that can be practically self-sustaining. In a society with so many resources, how can we not be meeting people's minimum needs?

Not as fast as yesterday. I'm disappointed with my pace as I check my watch for the last time. The part of me that wants to PR every time is shaking its head.

I walk to the parking lot, my watch says "job well done!" I put my results in my dictation, and head home.

## Day Four results
Weight: 244
Miles: 2.76
TOF: 37 minutes, 1 second
13:27 average pace

## My Watch is a Jerk.

My Nike Sportswatch gives me reminders every once in a while. "Are we going running?" and "Can't wait," as well as after-run encouragement: "Good job!" or "New record!"

But if you haven't run in a few days, it starts to sound a tiny bit sarcastic. It reminded me "Are we going running today?" (it's been 4 or 5 days), and when I clicked "okay" it responded with "Way to keep at it."

Way to keep at it? Are your tiny circuits judging me, dude? You want a piece of me, you insulting tiny timepiece?

Way to keep at it.

Screw you, watch.

## 5. "IF THIS WAS EASY, THEY'D CALL IT YOUR MOM." – SIGN AT MARATHON

I'm very sore, both in my legs and back. I don't think it was the running, I think it was the half-hour of lugging flagstones to the back of my house. This will not only test my resolve, it will test my body's ability to heal itself.

I am thinking about some of life's great questions this morning:

Would you rather be so smart you know everything, or perfectly happy?

Invisibility or flight?

Why has Karl survived for so many seasons on *The Walking Dead*?

In this frame of mind, I'm thinking running might be interesting, even though I might have to start my stretch routine with an Ibuprofen. Oh, by the way, I don't have a stretch routine. And the answers, obviously, are: "Happy," "Flight," and "kill off that character already."

After a job interview at a health club where they tell me I'm overqualified to be the assistant manager, I head over to a flat area of the Interurban trail for my run. Of course I'm overqualified. I just thought it would be fun to work in a health club.

I feel like I need a break, a visit to the country where I can reflect in the woods, like Henry David Thoreau. Will running become my daily "Walden"? I have no damned idea. All I can say it that I'm frustrated and I'm going to go run it off.

"I'm here to chew bubble gum and Run. And I'm all out of bubble gum."

I've chosen the Interurban trail. That's my jam.

When I told my wife this, she said "you're going to run in that sketchy area?"

Yes.

It's an eighteen-mile bike path from Everett, to Edmonds. I'll be running a piece in the lovely non-historic neighborhood near where we used to live. An area I call "The Heart of Darkness." This is the neighborhood we moved out of so our kids wouldn't have to go to *that* school, you know, the one no one wants to go to and is surprised to hear anyone still goes there, it's so awful. Yeah, that one. Every school district has that school, which shall not be named. They whisper of it in dark circles.

It's reasonably flat, it's pretty straight, and I'm running angry. So I don't really care who's on it. I dare ya.

The bike trail parallels I-5. I start out really fast and have to remember to slow myself back down, from my blistering nine-minute pace to a more normal pace I can sustain. Like the speed of honey.

It may be more and more important for us, as density increases in urban areas, to find those "Walden" moments, where we can be Henry David Thoreau and find our solitude and peace. Yoga, meditation, running. I've decided to give running a try at this because I loved it so much in my youth, so perhaps I can get back to that.

When my wife ran the Portland Marathon, someone held up a sign as she neared the finish line. My favorite sign of all time:

"If a marathon was easy, they'd call it your mom"

I love that. Always good to have a chuckle on the course. You know what? This run seems easier, despite my soreness. Maybe running angry is the key. Or maybe "easy" or "hard" isn't the issue, it's how you approach it. Forget easy. Just do it. That aphorism doesn't quite work if we go back to the "your mom" reference, but the point is clear: make the run your own, and get out of it what you can. Forget "easy" and "hard" – know that it's not going to be a glorious prance through space. It's probably not going to be "easy" – it's just going to be whatever you can handle. Your job is just to handle it.

Scott Jurek talked about random thoughts being the enemy of a distance runner. There are a lot of ways to perceive the idea of "clarity," and it dawns on me that my idea of it is wrong. We may not be chasing a state in which you have all these "epiphanies," or your thoughts are clear and concise. Rather, Jurek was referring to a clear mind, free of encumbrances. That may be my best realization yet, that I have been thinking about running all wrong – it isn't easy, or hard, it just IS. On your clearest moments, you're not tapped into the font of all knowledge, you're just empty and running.

It's the sixteen minute mark and I'm turning around. Looks like a slight uphill on the way back. Funny how when you're running downhill slightly it's difficult to tell, but when you're running uphill slightly whoooa nelly you know it.

One of the best finishes I ever had on a run was when I was running Big Gulch on the sidewalk back. There is a sidewalk crossing, and a truck slowed down, so I nodded and crossed. Before I was through he hit the gas and almost hit me! So I did the customary yelling at a window as the driver sped off. Texting? Stupid? Who knows. I finished that run angry and it felt fantastic, a slight charge of adrenaline fueling the finish as I bit my lip angrily.

At this year's New York Marathon the winner Wilson Kipsang was elbowed badly by the second place finisher, who tried to push ahead with about a half-mile to go. Kipsang glared at him. I mean glared, a look I know well because my wife glares like Kipsang. Kipsang had words, which could very well have been "oh, it's like that, is it?" and sprinted for the finish. He won handily. It was awesome to see. Run mad. Run harder.

Today's run brought to you by the saying: "Whatever doesn't kill you, makes you stronger."

26 minutes.

I slow down to a crawl, but keep running without stopping. I go past a man by the side of I-5, who doesn't see me because I am coming from behind him. He's strewing the trash from his backpack on the path. WTF is wrong with people?

28 minutes. I'm still running.

Isn't it amazing how the human will can be indomitable? How you can go through so much crap in your life and your mind responds by getting stronger? That's part of what I'm searching for. Setting a goal means you have to put yourself out there, on the line, and sometimes you need to do that just to say you did it. Forget the consequences, just put yourself out there and live without fear. 30 minutes. Booyah.

It's a good run.

## Day Five results
Weight: 242
Miles: 2.77
TOF: 30 minutes, 3 seconds
10:50 average pace – yeah baby!
503 kcal

I've been thinking about this all wrong. Running isn't about finding a happy place. Everything else can be so crappy. Running isn't a happy place – it's a way to get away from the crappy places everywhere else. Running is a way of working that stuff out, taking it out on the road, metaphorically punching someone in the face. It's a way to assert yourself that is solely about YOU. That's as important as anything, finding that place where it's just you and the road. That's the walk in the woods. That's Walden. Not some solitude that has to be away from people, or create magic thought-fairies in your mind. It's just you, dealing with your junk in the moment. Today, that's what I've discovered running can be for me.

## Are Runners Grown-up Superheroes?

Some part of me thinks that people who choose to run, over and over again in life, are heroic. I mean, you're basically saying "this hurts, but bring it ON!" It's rather brave to get out and punish your body for no other reason the slight hope to stave off age and disease for a little longer.

As you can tell, I'm still not really buying into the "Running is fun!" idea, which seems like running hired an excellent marketing team but no one is buying it. The "running is fun" crowd are probably the same people that believe that driving a certain car makes you sexy, or wearing a certain Brand of jeans makes you look hot. It ain't necessarily so.

Running is a diaper. Not exactly fun, but it's an effective way to deal with crap.

Still, the whole running thing is rather heroic, and the older you are the more impressive it is to us laypeople, those who lose cats up trees and are so pleased to have Superman retrieve them, or are effusive in our praise when you, Catwoman, trip up a purse-snatcher with your catarang and retrieve it for us little old ladies.

Catarang?

Well, whatever. Running is impressive to people who don't run in the same way Catwoman's assistance is impressive to the little old lady. Every run is a fight to a non-runner, like trying to will ourselves to fly without having an ounce of that gift.

There was a show in the 1970's called The Greatest American Hero. It was about a guy that found a superhero suit that gave him powers, but he lost the directions to the suit. Every takeoff and landing was about a 50/50 chance of failing, crashing, looking stupid. People who run effortlessly are to us slow slugs what the Greatest American Hero is to Superman. I mean, kudos and all, it's definitely impressive and we wish we could join you fighting crime, but we're not even sure we can make it to the scene of the crime without complete disaster.

We revere heroes in life as people who do things that aren't required of them, putting themselves into harm's way to help others. Soldiers, firemen. Runners are personal heroes, who wear their bodies down training themselves to be stronger, faster, fitter. That's a brand of heroism.

<I wave goodbye to Superman as he streaks off into the sky>

"Go get em, Supes!"

## 6. "IF AT FIRST YOU DON'T SUCCEED, TRY, TRY AGAIN. THEN QUIT. THERE'S NO USE IN BEING A DAMNED FOOL ABOUT IT." - W.C. FIELDS

My 12:30 time running two miles, lo those many years ago, was no accident. I trained for it by running a five-to-seven mile run every other day for twelve weeks, at speed I had never run at before or since. It definitely had a cost.

I was in advanced training at the Army base in Fort Sill, Oklahoma, and I remember waking up at zero dark thirty, getting our linens off of our beds, and shambling downstairs for PT formation. We would wait for them to call us into line. We always had a few minutes before that happened, so people generally made good use of that time by sleeping on the side of the stairwells, on a curb, anywhere where you could sit and put your head on your hands and rest. With white sheets draped over us, it looked like a bunch of silent ghosts loitering in a haunted barracks.

We'd run in formation, which is not the easiest way to run. A pothole was a deathtrap – you didn't see it coming unless the guy in front of you held up his hands as a signal. Running in formation also changed the way people ran, and the whole group was prone to the "slinky effect," where a few guys lag for only a few seconds, but you have to run like crazy to make up time. The problem is exacerbated on down the line, so there were many times where it seemed like you suddenly had to run a city block at your fastest pace to catch up with everyone who was running at a normal pace. Just like a slinky.

But the pace was never normal unless you were at the front of the line. Usually I was near the back. I spent basic training running in the "average" group of runners. I wasn't placed into the slow group, the

"Turtles," but I wasn't in the fast group either, the "Rabbits."

I thought I could be a Rabbit – at that time the average group's runs seemed kind of easy. We had a choice, so one day I fell into formation in the Rabbit line. It was a big deal for me, but no one else knew. I was a ninja rabbit. Off we went, running around base at what seemed like breakneck speed. I fell back from the group during the run. I caught up frantically. I fell back again at around mile three, and I knew I was done. I went back to the middle group for the next run, and kept with that group throughout the rest of Basic Training. As I recall, at the end of Basic Training my two-mile time was somewhere respectable, around 14:15. I thought I could do better.

When I got to Advanced Training, I decided I would try again. Early in that thirteen-week period, I also made the decision to join the fast group. This is key: I decided that I would stick with it. I persevered.

It was unbelievably hard. Some guys who turn out for the Army are extremely fit. I was running with those guys. We ran like heck, in the early early morning, singing cadence with our flashlights in hand. Darkness, song, footfalls. It's surreal to think about this time, finishing runs last of the three groups, not because we were slow, but because we ran so much farther than other groups, the sun just breaking as we hit the barracks to shower and get our BDUs(battle dress uniforms) on for a day of class, learning to fix radios.

The results were great on me, however. Helped to lean out my body. At a time when I was already 185 pounds, I developed more muscle because running toned me as our pushup and sit-up routines every other day built muscle mass.

I really wanted to do well on the final run. I wasn't the fastest runner in the group by a wide margin, but I knew if it was just two miles I could really put the hammer down and nail it.

Way to mix a metaphor, right?

As the run started, a one mile loop(we would run twice around) circling a large training area, I set an aggressive pace for myself. One I didn't think I could maintain. I was right. It was too fast. Still, I stuck with it and pushed as hard as I could. I'm sure my second mile was probably a minute slower than the first, but you don't get a 6:30 average by going slow at any time. It was very gratifying to me. Though I didn't get the maximum score(I recall at the time it was 11:54 to max it), I was very happy to have accomplished this feat. My fastest time EVER, and still my record by a longshot. If I look at my watch for pace during a run today, I can hit a 6:30, but I can't maintain that for long at all. I'm not getting any younger.

# Hulk takes a test

Yesterday I ran angry. Being angry has served me well in my life. During the same training period at AIT, we were tested every week on our knowledge of the subject matter taught. The subject matter was fixing radios. I know, it was exciting, thanks for noticing that. They posted the scores from the tests every week, and we were told at the beginning of training that if we were the top in the class on the tests, we would earn the title "Distinguished Honor Grad" at the end of training and get a commendation from a colonel. Due to a snafu with me being in the National Guard and on something called "split" training, my scores didn't show up for the first nine weeks of training. At the time, when they posted our scores it was a big deal for some of us, and the leader every week was a Private First Class named Kemper. I remember this because I hated that guy. He had a high, whiny voice, and he was the braggart of the class. You know the type, the guy who would dominate a conversation but didn't really have anything to add to it. I took an immediate dislike to him when I met him. He was leading the boards for nine straight weeks until my scores showed up on week tied. We were practically tied, but I had a slight edge with only three more weeks of testing.

He saw the scores and shrugged: "It's not really important to me anyway."

If he had said "wow, nice job Markey," it would have been different. Being flippant about it made me angry, because we both had worked hard at our scores, and we both knew it. If we, in our youth, had been able to shake hands and get to "may the best man win," then it would have been a friendly competition, and who knows how it would have ended.

Saying "It's not really important to me anyway" ticked me off. And as you know by now, I perform really well when I am angry. I guess I can relate to the Bill Bixby/Lou Ferrigno show "The Incredible Hulk" from the 1970's:

"Don't make me angry. You wouldn't like me when I am angry."

*turns into Hulk*

The Class was twenty or so Army guys, so no one really studied outside of class. I resolved to study hard, reviewing the information we had to cement the lessons. Everyone did the bare minimum in class, but I resolved to learn more and focus my attention. I nearly aced each of the last three tests. My lead grew slightly over Kemper each week. At the end of the training period, I was awarded the Distinguished Honor Graduate.

I played Angry. I won.

For today's run, I want to try something different, despite the angry success of yesterday. I want to run to our local donut shop and back. It was about twenty minutes away. I'll reward myself with a donut, and trot home.

It's a chilly run. I have my hat and gloves on and the wind blows right through my technical shirt. This is just running on the sidewalk with a few crossings along the way.

I'm surprised how my body has held up so far. I dreaded the soreness of this activity, and I thought by now my feet would be very sore and my muscles would start to break down. So far that is not the case, although my total mileage to date is relatively low. Maybe my body is adapting to this change in my running habit.

I feel almost, dare I say it, "spry."

I guess I dared say it.

It's very overcast and windy so I have extra praying to the gods of TomTom before my run can officially begin – about a one-third of a mile worth of walking, to be precise. That's a reference to my watch, of course. Always waiting on the danged watch.

I really try to start out slow today. That's made easier by a big hill on the sidewalk at the point where I start running, but I'm thinking about how awesome yesterday was, and how successful I was running slow to "catch my wind." I know it sounds stupid to point this out, but I am one of those guys that is oddly competitive, and this is a situation where being competitive doesn't help you at ALL. That may be why people complete marathons when they are older: they develop the patience needed to train for it. It's really sad to have to point this out to myself over and over again. I want to RUN, and speed feels really good.

So I creep up the hill and around the corner, probably a thirteen minute pace, just plodding along. It levels out so I can increase my pace a bit, but after the first half-mile, the wind kicks up to a whistle and pushes against me, slowing me further. The wind is your mom when you are driving and she brakes the car, slowing me down. I can't just brush off mom nature, so I tolerate it and keep pushing. I will get the wind at my back on the way down, so there's that to look forward to.

This is probably the point in the book where you young'ns are looking at my times and thinking "man, this guy is SLOW!" Ah, just you wait, grasshopper. Your time will come. You'll begin to slow. It's a fight, isn't it, to retain our health and our presence as we age. It's a fight to even get outside sometimes. I'm proud of the work I've done so far, even six days in.

It's pretty exciting to look at five or six days and realize that I'm creating what I set out to create. How often do we set goals that require us to do something for six days consecutively? That is a lesson in goalsetting. It doesn't matter what the goal is. You're either in an upward spiral in your self-image because you're working at attaining it, or you begin a downward spiral because you're moving away from it. You're either green and growing, or ripe and rotting. Even a tiny daily goal that you can make progress towards will help you build personal momentum.

I get close to the donut shop, and turn around. I'm *not* stopping for a donut. It's another old motivational trick I used to use on myself when I made sales calls. You build in a reward for yourself that you'd like, but sometimes you don't really feel like having the reward when you get to the place the goal is attached to. Sometimes it feels better to keep moving. There's nothing wrong with it. You still have the accomplishment of getting to where you wanted to, but you don't have to experience the reward all the time.

Smiley face emoji. Winky face emoji. Devil face emoji.

I'm on the downhill track on the way back to my house. It's a decent run, one of the smoothest so far. Am I getting stronger? Look up, look around, I keep reminding myself.

I take a long-cut through the park at 92nd street. I stop to clear a branch that has fallen across the path. I'm not setting any records for time as I coast into my neighborhood and towards my street, but I'm proud of my efforts and that I am actually doing this. Pro tip: if you start running on a 30-day challenge like this, keep a log. I'm really getting a charge out of seeing how I'm doing every day.

"Crowd Goes Wild" My watch says.

## Day Six results

Weight: 242 – holding strong at my pre-experiment weight. Ha.
Miles: 2.8
TOF: 30 minutes, 17 seconds
10:48 average pace
509 cal

## 7. "SOMETIMES I WRESTLE WITH MY DEMONS. SOMETIMES WE JUST SNUGGLE."

I really am experiencing a change in mood. It's fascinating to think about how this little experiment may be changing the way I think about myself. As you go along in life, you feel like you are becoming immune to such drollery, such mundane inspiration. Apparently, I'm not. Each day I seem to be gaining in confidence, and I was reasonably confident to begin with.

Mark Twain said "All you need is ignorance and confidence, and success is sure." Here's to being stupid for as long as I can.

I'm waiting for the other shoe to drop, really. It's going swimmingly well(where did THAT saying originate?), but I've had some satisfying runs of late. At some point, I know I'm going to hit a bit of a wall. I know that every person in every sport hits a personal obstacle at some point, and there's no way every run can continue to be awesome. So is my mood reflective of progress towards my goal, or the fact that my runs have been pretty good?

One of my favorite books is David McRaney's *You are Not so Smart*. McRaney likes to explore how we fool ourselves and how we fool others, often unintentionally. He talks about things like cognitive dissonance, confirmation bias, and the "Benjamin Franklin Effect."

One unintentional way our beliefs operate is the Anchoring principle. We have to have a source of comparison to form many of our beliefs, and oftentimes our first judgment lingers and biases our later perceptions. It's a kind of "first impression" for the brain. If someone tells us a pair of shoes is $250, and then we discover they are on sale for $180, the anchoring principle helps establish how much of a value those shoes are. It's difficult to get back to the idea that $250 is a ridiculous price in the first place.

I know this.

More to the point, my wife knows this. We've had discussions about this. But Mrs. Imelda Marcos insists she's *saving* so much she couldn't resist. The statement "You wouldn't believe how much I saved" is the starting point for many marital discussions about money, isn't it?

I believe we anchor our self-image in much the same way. We hold on to our beliefs about ourselves regardless of new information. It's hard to shake the specters of our past beliefs. There are things we feel we are capable of, and there are things we think we are not capable of. So when we read of Dean Karnazes' incredible story of how he started running by taking off for a 30-mile run in his underwear at age 30, our first reaction is "I could never do that."

Why not?

I mean, I'll admit to you that I don't plan on running 30 miles in my underwear anytime soon. But that doesn't eliminate the possibility that I might be able to undertake and complete such a thing.

We need a grand experiment, sometimes. We need to shake off our limits and think about new ones. Then we need to act on those impulses to push ourselves to where we need to get to.

Dean Karnazes is a ridiculous example due to his crazy lactate tolerance. It's like he's the Secretariat of Ultra-Marathoners. He's a freak. Still, sometimes, you have to be bold. As Dean says, be audacious. If, in your life, being audacious means lacing up for a two mile walk every day, then so be it. There are people who would kill to be able to walk. It's your body and your own definition of audacity.

I'm going out for my audacious 30 minute run now.

Big Gulch. I'm feeling Big, so why not challenge that.

Day seven! Today's weather is absolutely beautiful. As awful as it's been over the last week, you're probably asking "Why would you live near Seattle?"

A day like today is why.

The Poet Laureate of Seattle has to be the Cartoonist" The Oatmeal," and he put this on his Facebook page:

"Jesus RollerBlading Christ it's super nice in Seattle today!" *Picture of Jesus rollerblading on a rainbow*

It's a crisp, clear fall day with lots of leaves on the ground. It's just stunning. Pine trees, mountains – it's definitely why people live here. I take it easy for the first few minutes, then pause to get a couple pictures of the vista of Puget Sound, Whidbey Island to our west at the top of the first hill.

It's another day where I have to will myself to slow down, because I just want to RUN. I want to fly down the hill. Is that my problem this whole time? Not that I don't like running, but that I can't run fast enough to enjoy it? The unanswered questions remains around the subject of focus.

Is it that
1) When I focus I have a better run, or
2) Running leads to better ability to focus, or
3) Focus isn't the idea at all, but "clear-mindedness" IS?

I have to say that on day seven I am a lot less vested in these questions. I just don't care about the runner's high that much right now. I have committed to this exercise for 30 days, and whether or not I have some psychedelic magic shroom experience as a result of running two miles a day is really not the point.

I make it up only the first hill before I feel compelled to stop. I feel good, and I think my run time is okay. I'll just keep going.

One minute walk break. This run follows a much more typical pattern for me: run up one hill, a little walk break. Run up the next hill, another walk break.

Up one hill... down the other side... Up one hill... down the other side...

A lot of walk breaks today.

I run through the smelly part of the run, not running angry, not towards reward. It seems to me this run is kinda blasé. I need to kick myself in the butt to get this going. You know, it would be really helpful if a bear jumped out of the woods and started chasing me right now. That is a memo from the "careful what you wish for" department. That would help my time though, wouldn't it?

It's amazing how few runner's I've seen on my runs so far. I just passed a 60 year old man gutting it out, and I can't help but think to myself "yeah, brother, you keep on with it!"

I dare a glance at my watch – my time is not too bad, so I must be doing something right. I make the decision to further challenge myself and go up what my son's Cross-country team calls "Hell Hill." My son told me last year that rumor has it that no one has <u>ever</u> made it up Hell Hill without stopping.

Turns out, the next year I found out that rumor was completely false. People on the cross-country team had run up Hell Hill without stopping regularly. I didn't hit snopes.com to verify it, so I guess that one's on me.

A young man passes me coming from the other side of the gulch, asking for directions. I point him to the same place I'm going, up Hell Hill. And look at him. He's got his school backpack on and his jeans, and up he goes running up it. I guess there's no excuse for me now, is there. I run up behind him.

Spoiler alert: I don't run up Hell Hill. Even a walk up a steep hill is a good workout.

At least, that's what I'll say as I cry myself to sleep tonight.

I take off running again at the top, having a bit of an energy boost from my break. "Finish strong," I say to myself. Yeah, what you do is you walk two point-nine miles and run the last point-one miles. Finish strong. Always finish in front of your neighbors too.

Ahh, blessed flatness, how I've missed you. My music shifts into a breakbeat rhythm and I pick up the pace.

I pass the young man who ran up the hill on the flat. He says "nice, man!" as he watches me pass. Then he turns it again and passes me. I stay up with him until I turn on my street.

I have a strong finish – whenever I'm finishing this run back to my house there's only one small hill and a bit more downhill, so the run almost always feels breezy on the way home. I felt strong at the end, but struggled in the middle.

## Day Seven results: "Nice finish" says my watch.

Weight: 242. Same old same old.
Miles: 2.8
TOF: 34 minutes, 17 seconds
12:10 average pace
513 cal
Mood: Thank God that's done.

## I am only HALF-crazy.

My wife talked me into a half-marathon about seven years ago. Hey, we had only been married a couple years. I still had that newlywed glow. We ran with our friends, who I will call Tessa and Taylor. Tessa likes running and is rail-thin, but Taylor is not particularly fit. I think he likes his beer. I like Taylor.

It was a hot day, over 80 degrees. I trained, even completing a nice nine mile run a week or so before. I was ready!

No, I wasn't.

The course started along the Sammamish River Trail and wound up through the University of Washington's Bothell campus. Up, up, up. In the heat. It was brutal.

The trail wound down and curved back on to the Burke Gilman, but by mile seven I was cramping badly. For the next six miles I shuffled, then hobbled as the cramping was too bad. I finished in around two hours and 40 minutes. I was miserable. My wife passed me at around mile ten. Tessa passed me too. Guess who was the fastest in our foursome?

Taylor. The fat guy. Kicked our butts. Isn't that the way of it? He even looked better than all of us afterwards, sweaty but almost fresh, like he could do it again. Dork.

The funny part, in an almost Friday the thirteenth kind of way, was my self-talk. By the time the cramping started, my internal monologue was dramatically different than it was at the beginning of the race. I started the race confidently:

"You can do it!"

"Keep it going!"

After a few miles, I started to say things like "Wow, hot day," and "We're still climbing?"

Then my inner monologue got worse.

"Why would I subject myself to this?!"

"Whose stupid idea was this?"

"This is the dumbest damn thing I have ever done in my life."

"&*%$@!"

I finished. It wasn't pretty. It was really really not pretty.

The whole event was pretty comical – in retrospect. How my self-talk plummeted into hatred. It didn't have to, but man, I was an unhappy camper at the end of that run.

Come to think of it, that was the last time I saw Taylor.

# 8. "NO SANE MAN WILL DANCE" – CICERO

It's a Saturday, so after my son's soccer game I hit the trail at another Everett park, Narbeck Wetland Sanctuary.

If you have children that like playing sports, and you are struggling to figure out how and when to work out. Good news! The answer is in front of you. Sometimes my kids have to be at games a half hour early for "warmups," so guess what? That's a great time for the adults to warm up too. It amazes me to see parents that bring out their camping chairs and sit on their butts for an entire game. Get out of that chair. Run a lap around the field. Do a couple pushups, would that be so bad? Do we need to watch every move our children make? I have done pull-ups on nearby monkey bars many times. I don't do many. But I do them.

Standing is better than sitting. I don't understand why people plop themselves in a chair to watch their kids get in activity. What kind of a message is that sending? Do we think our children are going to grow up and be active if our job as adults is sitting in a chair watching them do things? Adults complain about how they don't have any time to work out. Guess what? If we have kids, we do!

It's very exciting to watch your kids play at game time, but if you're struggling with this issue, isn't your health and fitness as important as your kids' health and fitness? Heck, you could be crazy innovative and just do a couple jumping jacks on the sidelines. Are we so worried about how we'll look that we're unwilling to do that? Get active on the sidelines, moms and dads.

I'm starting out today just on the east side of Boeing. Narbeck Wetland Sanctuary is just off Seaway Boulevard in Everett, and is quite literally across the street from the main entrance to the Boeing plant. It's another gorgeous day in Puget Sound, a cloudless morning, blue sky and sunshine. It's still 50 degrees, but clear and crisp, like a fall apple. Perfect running weather.

Eight days in, I'm starting to get a bit of a sinking feeling. I'm concerned that I may be able to complete this challenge and have little "net" result. I'm not that sore – more on this in a minute – so at the end I may not be any more "fit" than when I started. I may not have lost any more weight. I may not love running. I may have accomplished nothing more than get out and wear down a pair of shoes. Yay. The competitive part of me thinks "what's the point of that?" and I wonder if I should increase my mileage a bit to *really* challenge myself. I know in doing so I risk injury, I risk taking myself out of the experiment entirely. I'm torn in this idea, but at the same time if I am only just a little bit sore every day – which I am very surprised at – but if I am only a tiny bit sore, then I might have set my bar too low. My plan is to give it another week before I change anything. Obviously I want to be successful in this challenge, but I'd like to have something to show for it. I'd like to lose a few pounds. I'd like to feel like I'm getting a tiny fraction of a bit faster.

I want to experience "I ran for 30 days and I learned this." "I ran for 30 days and saw marked gains in my leg strength." "I ran for 30 days and learned so much about myself." "I ran for 30 days and it was a life-changing experience." I became this, I grew in this way. I developed the ability to solve quadratic equations in my head, I don't know. Something. I guess I'm starting to question why I'm doing this, and I don't have any answers. Finding answers is omnipresent in my mind as I pull into the Sanctuary's parking lot.

So far, it's "I ran for eight days and it was meh."

As I talk to my sons about my challenge, do you know what their response is? Meh. That's right. As Dad takes on a new challenge for himself, I am met with a rousing cheer of "hey-let's-go-play-more-xbox." I think they understand implicitly that while it's a challenge to put on my shoes and go take my slow ass out there for a run, it's not audacious. It's tedious.

Tedious. That may capture, in a word, why I fell out of love with Running. It became tedious. I discovered a bicycle. Running became the slower way to move. It became work. The essence of running became training to get better, and that is so boring.

So here I am out here on day eight for a run, trying to bring the sexy back.

At the Sanctuary I spend a few minutes looking at the guideposts and signs. I love reading that Narbeck has an interpretive shelter and an interpretive trail. I love the word "interpretive" because it always reminds me of interpretive dance.

I've been in this park before, but I ran the perimeter and didn't notice the crazy concrete shelter. It's like a giant zoo viewing area. It has a couple large portholes as windows. It's covered in moss. A Hobbit-house, I think. Okay, that's not really what I think as I walk inside it. I half expect to see homeless people. It's empty.

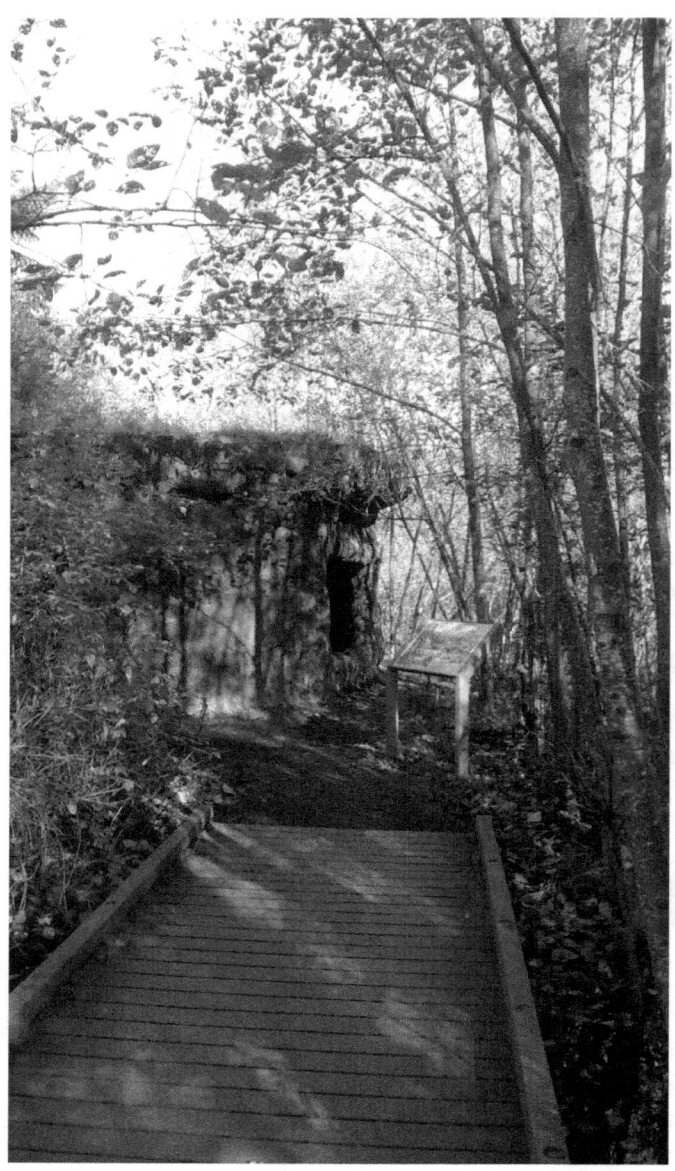

I do have a bit of soreness in my hips, which is weird. My wife has some cryptic yoga stretch she does to work that out, but I'm not used to hip soreness and I can't mimic this Bhagavadgita or whatever pose very well, so it's lingering.

I'm starting on the road next to Narbeck and across from Boeing, mostly because it's sunny and I'm still a bit cold. This isn't a big trail so I'll have to wind around it a time or two to get my 30 minutes on 48 acres of land. I want some warmth. In Washington, you take warmth whenever it presents itself in the fall.

This feels like an easy run, even from the start. I don't have a prescribed trail, a defined start and finish, so that's a bit freeing, isn't it? Running unrestrained by those conditions. Real runners talk about how much they hate out and backs, at least in part for these reasons:

You go out and stop at a prescribed point, so you have an exact turnaround "limit," and

You see the same stuff coming back as you did going out.

It's purely psychological, of course.

The feeling of not having particular markers or an area you're running to or back from is relatively freeing in this way. Run as far as you want, loop around, and if it's not enough running, then do some of it again.

Narbeck Sanctuary is a lot different than some of the Washington wetlands I've run through. Typically, a wetland is a large grassy marsh with water in it. It has waterfowl and teems with life underwater, but it's flat and not many trees grow in that muck. Narbeck has birch tree stands throughout, so you have large stands of water with birch trees. It's really open-feeling and you have good visibility into the forest, which is fairly rare in Washington. The blackberries have not taken over this space. East of the Cascades has more open spaces, but the forests here are dense and sometimes impassable.

I find myself running along a well-designed walkway made of plastic decking material. This is the "Interpretive" part of the trail so I try out my best interpretive dance moves as I run. I call my artistic results "Spring", "The Birch Tree Speaks", and "Angry Duck."

I go back to the outside of the perimeter of the park. I try not to think about how I look as I mosey along at what I will charitably call a running pace. This way madness lies. You start worrying about how you look doing things and all of a sudden you're buying better clothes when it really doesn't matter. You're going to get hot and sweaty anyway.

I probably look just like my professional picture. Take that picture, replace my face with the face of a man who looks like he's going to say something abjectly stupid, mouth half open, a grimace that says he is mildly uncomfortable, add a bunch of flop sweat, a glazed over look in my eye and there ya go. It's practically the same thing. *Nobody looks good running.*

I look at my watch as I come back out on the road. I stop for a walk break at the eighteen minute mark. Feels like a pretty good run.

I find myself dictating less and running more, which I believe is another good sign that I am able to clear my mind and focus on the "spirit" of a run.

Looping back through the parking lot at 23:00, I make a bold – bold, I say! – decision to make another full loop around the Sanctuary, thereby extending my time by several minutes. I also invite myself again to FINISH this experiment. I've started a lot of things in my life, but I haven't finished nearly as many. Ask my wife and the 30 unfinished home projects.

This, I will finish. So proclaimeth me in the middle of my run.

Now I realize I have trapped myself on the interpretive trail, which doesn't appear to have another way out besides the loop I've already run. I'm doomed to interpretive dance forever! Oh, nope, there are the stairs up to the other trail.

If you don't want to stop for walk breaks when running, run where there are many people. If you're running on a trail and you stop next to people, that seems a bit stalker-y, so you keep going. If you stop in front of them, that's weird, so you keep going. If you stop behind them and start panting for breath, that's definitely weird, so you keep running. Better to run past them. Really important running etiquette tip.

I have run today entirely without my music. I took my headphone off so I could hear a bit more of nature. I could hear the cadence coming out of my headphones. It was rather peaceful to run this way.

I'm break my rules with ½ mile to go and look at my watch. I look at my pace and try to better it. It's 11:20. Let's see if I can improve on that in my final time.

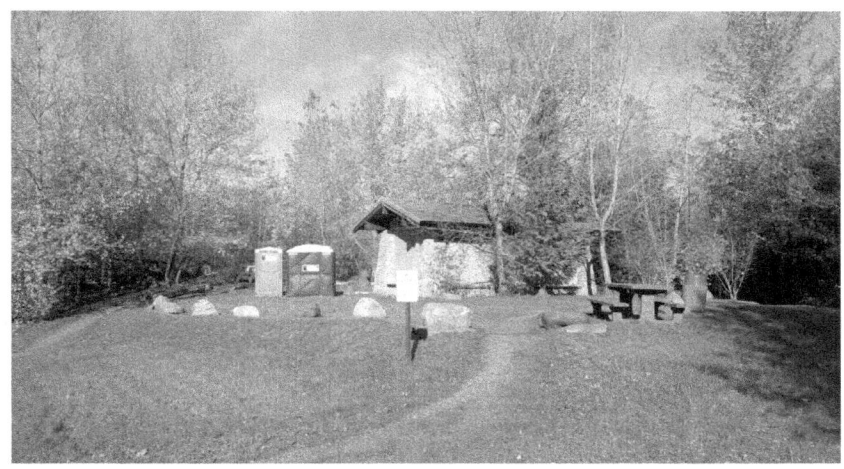

I am proud of the composition of this photo, with the fall foliage, the picnic table, the no-smoking sign at center and the porta-potties. The porta-potties right next to the bathroom building?

It occurs to me as I huff back to the parking lot that 11:20 isn't bad at all! An extra charge at the end nets me eight seconds on my average pace.

There I go with my competitive nature again. I just can't back off of it, can I?

## Day Eight Results:
Weight: 243
Miles: 3.13
TOF: 35 minutes, 3 seconds
11:12 average pace
568 cal
Attitude: Decent. I mean, hey, I'm not waxing poetic.

After my run today, I get a little frustrated. It's as if I'm expecting some transformational experience. I'm not forming a chrysalis here. I'm not a caterpillar metamorphosing into a danged butterfly. It's just running. It's not a damned spiritual awakening. To Luke Skywalker: "Stay on target. Stay on target."

## Running and Creativity:

I have a pretty good background in theater as part of my formal education(there's an oxymoron: "formal theater education"), and when I am running, or painting, playing music, it's the act of creation that is invaluable. It's something that comes solely from you, and the product is uniquely yours.

Running does have some similarities to the arts in that running is absolutely personal to you. It's your own experience. If you look at it that way, then you realize that since it's your own experience, there's no "right" way to do it, no "wrong" way. The key is doing it. The gift is the growth you experience doing it, not the product of your efforts.

We work out to help our bodies get in shape, but we neglect the idea that there is an inherent benefit to working with our minds, working out our minds, working on our minds. If you're starting a workout regimen, your goal may just be to look in the mirror and see your ripped self staring back. But it's also gratifying to experience the personal accomplishment that running represents. Kurt Vonnegut spelled this out clearly in his response to a class of schoolchildren who wanted him to visit. He declined the visit, but gave them this sage advice in a letter:

"Practice any art, music, singing, dancing, acting, drawing, painting, sculpting, poetry, fiction, essays, reportage, no matter how well or badly, not to get money and fame, but to experience becoming, to find out what's inside you, to make your soul grow."

I would offer to Mr. Vonnegut that exercise might have a similar effect on our psyche. What a lot of people don't realize is that doing "the arts" requires tremendous discipline. Running does too, and it's like the arts in that it's about what you can do. To make your soul grow.

# 9. "ONLY IDIOTS REFUSE TO CHANGE THEIR MIND" - BRIDGETTE BARDOT

I went to a running forum online yesterday(I did! Isn't that amazing?! Yay internet!) and looked up how people are doing with their runs. One woman says she runs at about a 21 minute mile pace. That IS very slow. I feel a bit of schadenfreude about that. Wow, that's slow.

Still, I'm not exactly a gazelle. It's popular on those forums for people to have a signature line on each of their posts that lists their PRs for different distances. I created mine:

"400 yards: frustratingly slow * 1 mile: slower than that * 5K: been there, sucked at that. Marathon: you have to be kidding"

No way am I competing with this group. It's really amazing how amazingly fast these amazing runners are. Amazing and depressing. At least I have the 21 minute miler to feel good about. Schadenfreude. I think that's why Honey Boo-boo was popular for a while.

Everyone is good for something, if only a bad example.

There are plenty people at every race that walk the entire thing. In fact, they won't shuffle into a run at any moment. No thank yew. These people are more than content to leave their egos at the starting line and slow-walk their way to success. I admire that, as do most runners, like author Joe Muldowney. They're not worried about how they look, and they are certainly not worried about their time. I'm not talking about the "4th annual Snohomish River Kiwanis Family Run/Walk" either. These are actual factual real 5ks with people who compete at the front and are finishing in under 20 minutes. That means that some of these cheetahs are finishing practically as the walkers cross the starting line. Get 'er done.

I posted a response to the 21-minute miler on the Runner's world forum. It's not about how everyone else is doing. I wrote:

"The journey is yours and yours alone."

Quick on the draw today. I arrive the prescribed 45 minutes early to my son's soccer game for his warmups. That allows me the prescribed 30+ minutes to go for a run. Well no time like the present!

We're in Sultan, Washington, east of my home and towards Stevens Pass, on a day that is rainy and 46 degrees. I stop at "Osprey" park, which looked to be a small park when I looked it up online. Look at that, the park sign says it has 2 miles of trail! Well, that's serendipitous. I don't hold my breath as I set my watch to sync up on a cloudy day, but it syncs up immediately. It's a sign!

Looks level, flat, right next to the Sultan River, so I just take off running.

The City of Sultan didn't mark this with any information on their website, so it's a hidden little gem of a park I've discovered. I go over a quaint little metal bridge crossing a creek that merges with the Sultan River. Rainy and wet, but beautiful. This season's rains are already taxing the River's maximum capacity. It might be in flood stage somewhere.

I've always maintained that there's something special about exercising when no one else is doing it. On a trail by yourself, early in the morning. Late at night. No one else is that dumb. It gives you a special feeling, knowing that YOU are that dumb. No one can take that away from you, that special feeling of how dumb you are.

I take a break after less than a mile. I'm gasping a little bit. I was pushing it. It was fun. Weird, huh? I'm using "fun" in a sentence that refers to running.

It used to be that all of my runs – such as they were – were all me sprinting out of the gate, and then walking. And then sprinting, and then walking. By "sprinting" I mean running at a seven or eight minute mile pace. Run, walk, rinse and repeat. I'd do that for 200 yards, a half a mile, MAYBE a mile, but never longer than that. It's back to that today. Total fail. It's like my brain thinks that if I run faster it will be over faster, and I can't convince it that I am running for time and not distance.

I come back to the park entrance for lap one and there is an old(~1988?) black Chevrolet Monte Carlo moving slowly around the parking lot, backing up, changing directions, like it's pacing. Idling, back and forth. I find myself wondering of course "who is that?" "what are they doing?" "why are they doing it?" I think about how women must feel in this situation. I'm a big guy. No one is going to mess with me unless they have a knife or gun and are desperate. There was a video recently that went viral about an actress who walked along the streets of

New York for ten hours, getting a lot of catcalls. I'm forced to think of the misogyny that still exists in our society. It was an interesting video, not because of what happened on it, which was really not much more than a bunch of guys being creepy and saying "hey Mami!" What was interesting about it was how people reacted. People's reactions to the video ranged from "men are jerks" to "she shouldn't be living in NYC if she doesn't want to be treated that way" and "they were just trying to compliment her."

And to be fair, it could be perceived as complimentary. Kinda. In an "I love objectifying YOU, baby" kinda way. In a Bill Cosby way. Okay, that might have been too soon.

If a compliment makes someone feel uncomfortable, it's not so much of a compliment, is it? It's an interesting issue – gamergate is going on right now too, and it's a tough thing to work out. It's a challenge being a woman, feeling threatened walking down the street. It's tough being a man figuring out how to treat women respectfully. You know what though? That's our job, fellas, to figure out how to treat each other respectfully, men and women. There was no respect in that video. There's enough trolling on the internet, it should never happen in real life like that. As a society, we have issues. So many are too stubborn to ever realize they are wrong.

Anyway, I swear this Monte Carlo was leering at me, but I'm back in the deep dark woods where it's safe.

I talked to my wife about running last night. She was confused as to why I made the distinction between the clear moments you have running and the idea-cornucopia moments. The Clarity and the Eureka. Why get hung up on distinguishing those things? "They are both reasons I run," she said. Both are wonderful. Isn't that a damnably healthy outlook. I'm trying to make a distinction between the two, trying to figure out which is more important, but both are equally valid. We can be inclusive. We don't have to be anti-Clarity or anti-Eureka. We don't have to be racist about running.

I'm struck by the same kind of intellectual snobbery in running forums. Everyone has their own judgments on speed, technique, and many are willing to derisively call people out as "hobby joggers" because their time is weaker. How indubitably lame. This is a personal journey. If you're too narrow to understand that a slow 18 minute running mile could be a victory for someone, then you, sir, should be reclassified as *homo lameitus*. The feelings we experience as Schadenfreude are nothing more than Trolling in our mind. Your personal journey may be faster, but it doesn't make it better, any more than a quick McDonalds burger is better than a slow, juicy steak. We admire speed too much. Me included. All journeys have value. It's your own personal journey to fitness, your own personal journey to your own insights, and who cares what judgment comes from those judgey judgers.

When it comes to the Clarity/Eureka distinction, one might not be possible without the other. Does clearing your mind lead to a burst of ideas? Or a burst of ideas might give way to a moment of silence in the brain?

Inventors have made use of this idea, and sociologists and psychologists suggest that being in an environment free from distractions can help inspire creativity. That might be exactly what we're talking about when we talk about getting "clarity" when running.

"You better lose yourself in the music, the moment, you own it, you better never let it go" – Eminem, "Lose Yourself"

19:00 through my "run" and I've done more talking to myself than anything else. Time to get it going.

Trailrunner's log entry: When running in the Pacific Northwest, always make sure to have a spare pair of shoes and socks in the car. You're probably going to step in a puddle. That is all.

25 minutes. Definitely slower today, owing to the fits and starts of running and walking. Still, I finish the run off by running onto the covered basketball court in the park and jumping up and down, "Gonna Fly Now" playing in my head, Rocky-style. No one else is in the park. My stalker car has left, thank goodness.

## Day Nine Results: "way to get out there"
Weight: 242
Miles: 2.58
TOF: 30.09
11:41 average pace
468 cal
Attitude: Well allrighty then.

## I Make the Cooking

Can I share a recipe of something that is actually healthy that I eat? Cold Oatmeal. I know, it's weird. I never knew I would grow up to become the guy that likes cold oatmeal. Please don't ruin my perfect recipe by using that nasty instant stuff. Quaker is fine, though. You don't have to use that gluten-free steel cut fancypants variety. I mean you can, but it's a bit much. Can you say "Oatmealkill?"

## Cold Oatmeal.

- Get some Oatmeal(Quaker). Probably like a cup or something. I'm no chemist.
- Fourteen Raisins.
- Cinnamon to taste, which there is no accounting for.
- Honey all over that mess.
- Milk, just to barely cover it all. If you put too little in your stuff will be dry and that's no good. Then you have to take a bit and hold it in your mouth until it moistens. That takes hours.

Put all stuff in a bowl. Make sure the bowl is big enough, but not ridiculously big, unless you are going to take pictures and want to go for a tiny human thing, in which case you will need an enormous spoon also. Put it in the fridge overnight. Yes, this requires forethought. I never said this would be easy! Some recipes take like eight hours in the crockpot or something, and you have to stir it. So I don't feel bad about it. The fact that there is advance prep needed legitimizes the recipe. Otherwise, it's just some lame placeholder in a book, but because it requires you to do something in advance that means it's a real recipe.

Vocabulary tip: if you want to impress your friends, use the word "gourmand" a lot to describe yourself. Just a random thought there, but free with purchase of this recipe.

Oh, and then eat the oatmeal. I am always surprised when recipes leave this part out, because it is the most fun part. The eating.

Serves: One. Might be you. Might not be you. I don't want to introduce the idea of the id, ego, concepts of other versus concepts of self, discuss about selflessness and get all philosophical here. It's just a recipe, calm down there Sigmund Freud.

# 10. "AS A MAN THINKETH IN HIS HEART, SO IS HE." – PROVERBS

It's a beautiful day today, and I'm going for a run with my wife. She's going about four miles on another sidewalk jog outside our home, but I'll turn around at some point and do my normal three miles. I feel privileged to be running with the master here, she's approaching a ten minute pace. Always something to aspire to for a noob like me.

I say we're running together, but not really. We start out together, that's our norm. Usually I go forward a bit too fast and then she passes me either while I'm still running, or, more frequently, a mile in when I'm slowing down and taking a walk break.

Oh crap, she's right behind me! - Be cool. *whistles*

My wife doesn't like running with me because I run so inconsistently, both in pace and frequency. Plus, running is her happy place. Thou must not enter the happy place of thy spouse. That's a law.

She's not competitive, and I am, so when we run together we do this odd jockeying for position thing. Not exactly the end of the NYC marathon, but we leapfrog each other constantly. I maintain that she is an entirely different runner when she gets in front of me than when she is behind me. There have been some times when she has a terrible run and doesn't seem to be able to get in front of me(usually that means I am having a great run). There are many more times when she gets in front of me and I don't see her until the run is over.

I'm proud I can run all the way up this hill today. It's only a half-mile out, but a challenging hill. That seems stronger for me.

The secret to running longer might just boil down to slowing down. My wife starts all her runs slow, but it seems painfully slow to me. My competitive nature gets the best of me, and I have to speed up, which gasses me. Right now I'm ahead of my wife, but she always has good negative splits. Mine are usually terrible – unless it's downhill. For those who want to get to longer distances while running, that could be some insight.

Up Mukilteo Speedway: as I turn the corner, I sneak a glance behind me. Nope, I haven't lost her, that's for darned sure.

It's impressive to me that some people can gain strength like that. They have to warm up for a mile or two. Warm up for a mile or two? That could be my whole run.

"Now what's up" (He says in his best Jerry Seinfeld impression) "with the people who talk while they run?"

I have run with friends like this, and it's crazy to me. They have so much breath left over, they can waste it on speech. I'm trying to make sure I don't asphyxiate.

Them: "So hey Tony, how's work going. I'm on a new project and it's a lot of fun. How have you been?"

Me: *Gasp* "Good."

Them: "I don't usually run this slow, but sometimes I like to slow it down a little. Have you been running much lately?"

Me: *Gasp* "Not." *Gasp* "Really."

What's worse is they talk in an absolutely normal voice. I'm sucking wind and they sound like they are sitting on a barstool sipping wine. If you could hear my dictation right now, you would know that I am taking regular breaths to gulp down more air. I even pause the microphone in the middle of a sentence sometimes. Anyway, those people are stupid.

I have a pretty good pace set for myself. I near the halfway point at the library. Out and back. Wooohoo.

I would be really impressed with myself, if I get a negative split this run. My pace is under 11:00. I high five my wife at the turnaround. I stayed in front of her!

The good news is I had that burst at the beginning and that was a half-mile uphill. A negative split is possible here since it's mostly downhill on the way back… if I can keep it going.

I do. I feel strong today. Was my goofy pace yesterday, with the walking and the sprinting, baby-interval training?

I go by a couple of City of Mukilteo employees that are happily cutting down dead branches from where they might land on the sidewalk. Their truck is blocking the path almost completely, but they are nice enough to not only stop their cutting, but make sure the branches are out of the way as I go around the truck and get back on the path. I smile and say "sucking diesel!" as I run by the last worker(in reference to the truck fumes I'm inhaling). He smiles and waves. He has earplugs in.

I'm also breaking my rule about not looking at my watch. It is such a good run, that I know nothing will stop me. I felt ups and downs this morning, but this run was consistently good, and I'm surprised. This is probably the first time on this experiment that I can say "I FEEL GOOD." I almost feel like a runner. It's wonderful, actually. I should tell my wife I need to "crash" her runs more often.

This has to be a negative split... and it is! I did it.

I reflect on the question "Have I had runs like this before?" the answer is yes. I have runs where it actually feels good to run. They are incredibly rare. Of the 30-50 times in a year where I run, I might have that twice. That's not an exaggeration. So every six months I feel good about a run. The rest is misery. It's that futile exercisey feeling. Those runs start with "this is going to suck," and end with "Well, at least I know I'm not dead." It helps to run a race of some sort, but that just feels like I'm putting lipstick on a pig.

Today's glorious run to Elysium happened pretty quickly by my own normal timescale, in a ten-day time-frame. I'm cautious. For all I know, this might be the only superfly yee-haw run of the experiment. I guess we'll see, but for today I own the victory.

### Day 10 Results: "High five"

Weight: 243
Miles: 2.86
TOF: 30 minutes, 10 seconds
10:32 average pace
500 cal

Attitude: Excellent. I would even Watch Bill and Ted again, that's how excellent. And that movie is terrible so you know I must be feeling good.

### Make a mess. Clean it up.

One of the problems with self-reflection is that it seems manic, at times, especially when viewed over days or weeks. You try to capture your own ups and downs, but it seems like you are on a mental rollercoaster. In a single day, the hours between your upbeat moments and your downtrodden ones disappear as you try to recall events. You remember the highs and lows, but risk sounding bi-polar when you recall them.

My office at home is an explosion of papers, stacked haphazardly across the room. I began a project today to clean off my desk. That meant I needed to go through some of my old files, some of which I haven't looked at in years. Once I go through my old files, I reasoned, I can go through the newer piles in my cabinet and file them. Then I can clear my desk.

So I make a mess before I clean it up. That's the idea.

So it is with my running challenge. I don't like running, so I made a plan to do it. Do it all the time. Make a mess of it. Make sure you don't like it by digging deep in your reserves of patience, swallowing whatever pride you have to make yourself a mess and hope by the end everything will be cleared up.

"…it would seem foolish, would it not, to adjust our lives to the demands of a goal we see from a different angle every day? How could we ever hope to accomplish anything other than galloping neurosis?" – Hunter S. Thompson

My hope-against-hope is that by day 30 I'll clear this up. By Day 30 I will have made sense of what seems like madness. Making sense means Clarity, right? There's that term again.

## 11. "THE TWO MOST COMMON ELEMENTS IN THE UNIVERSE ARE HYDROGEN AND STUPIDITY." – HARLAN ELLISON

"Congratulations! You are registered for the Amica Insurance Seattle Marathon 2014."

What a maroon. What a nincompoop. I can't believe I'm doing this on November 30th.

My wife suggested the other day that I might do the Seattle Half Marathon. That's thirteen miles – more than four times the length of my usual run.

"Ha, ha," I said.

The more I thought about it, the better it sounded. This should give you an insight into my intelligence level. I don't have any illusion that this won't be difficult. It will probably be a lot like being punched in the gut repeatedly for a few hours. However, I've been thinking about creeping up on mileage during this challenge since it's been going well. Registering for the half-marathon cures me of that disease immediately. The race is on November 30th, the very last day of the challenge. What better way to see if I'm gaining in strength? What better way to see if I can fall back in love with running? What better way to go out than with a bang?

The "bang" will probably be the sound of my Achilles and knee ligaments popping as they fall away from my body.

I would like to think that running for half an hour each day equals training, but I don't think there's a training book that says:

a) Running two or three miles per day will prepare you for 13.1 in ANY way, or

b) That running every day up to the race day is anything but a bad idea.

So I'm pretty much relying on genetics at this point. As I mentally count the number of fat relatives I have, the prospect of a terrible race on the 30th looms large.

Of course when I say "fat," I don't really mean that. I mean my relatives tend to be "gravity-challenged."

Today is Veterans Day, which means that I get to spend the day with my lovely children. They really are lovely. Lovely little bastards, I love 'em. They are in full pre-teen/teen mode, all three of them, so it's like bringing a bag of old jokes to a sarcasm festival every day. Oh, the eye-rolling. The backtalk. Fantastic.

We do have fun together. Today we're going to a park to play soccer. I'll take off from the park and do my run as they start playing soccer without me.

It's a beautiful clear day but it's COLD, blustery, the wind is whipping around and it feels like we live in Chicago. It will freeze tonight and its 37 degrees now. It's sunny and clear, so ask long as the wind doesn't pick up you're okay. If the wind picks up at all, it turns you into a popsicle.

We're at Kasch park nearby our house in the late afternoon. My children have decided they want to shoot goals for soccer, and so I'm going to run nearby. My plan is to take off and run to the back side of the park a half mile away, come back, run some more on the sidewalk. This is the most boring run I've ever conceived of.

I'm not going to worry about time at all. We'll see where we end up. I don't exactly have an "attack strategy" on this run. I'm just going to get out and move my legs, see what happens at the end of the day. Of course my kids want to press me into service to play soccer, which will be fun, but I have to get my run in first.

I start running to the back of the park. A weird and non-picturesque run. I might as well be in Arizona. No offense to my friends in Arizona; but you have to admit there's some boring stuff to see in the desert.

I run to the end of the park and work my way back, a whopping 8 minutes of work. Yeah, you heard me, it feels like work. Then I run around the soccer field they are playing on in circles, running back and forth from goal to goal while they play. It's a field big enough for nine year olds, so it's not very big. The sun goes down and the temperature begins to drop.

Every once in a while I end up with the ball as my kids kick it to me, or I kick a ball back from a nearby field. It reminds me of what I have always enjoyed: working out with a purpose. If you say "go grunt for a while," that never has any appeal for me. If you turn it into a game? That is a different story. I love playing basketball, but I'm terrible. I played soccer as a lad, but haven't since. Soccer is still an exercise, and I love the focus of playing a game.

It's twenty minutes before I give up my plan. Screw it. Running can be monotonous, but if you "gamify" it, then you can turn something boring into something exciting.

Run around for a while? Lame. Start keeping score with a point for a shot that goes in the net? Now you're talking.

If you gamify something, that becomes your focus. That's good and bad. I wouldn't expect to have moments of clarity, or even inspiration from that. Playing the game is entirely the focus. Yet, you develop a natural focus on the mechanics of the game, and you keep your body moving. That's rather the point, isn't it?

With an app called "Level me up," you can turn any activity into a game that gives you levels based on your proficiency. It's like turning an activity into a rewarding Role-playing-game activity to develop yourself.

At twenty minutes, I start running with the boys, playing soccer. Another boy joins us, who insists his nickname is Ronaldo, though his real name is Alex. He's around ten years old.

It strikes me now, as I play with my children, that I may have missed a larger point with this challenge. This is something I am famous for. Seeing the forest through the trees is remarkably difficult. The point is that Running is the activity, and how you get to it doesn't matter. Treadmill. Stairs. Sports. Trail. Who cares? My experiment is to see if I can fall back in love with running, not if I can learn to love Trail-running in particular, or that it has to be sidewalk, or that I even have to run for the entire time. I want to see if I can get back to loving the activity under any conditions, not under some artificial or sterile-seeming conditions that we sometimes create for ourselves adults.

A treadmill? I think a treadmill is a fine argument for gun control, because running on a treadmill makes me want to shoot myself.

Who cares what makes me run, as long as I run?

Still: it feels a bit like a cheat. Running with a purpose is so much more fun than running back and forth for little other reason than to challenge yourself. I let my watch run as I play with my kids.

At the end of the day, would I rather challenge myself with a ten minute mile, or play with my kids and achieve the same fitness level?

## Day 11 Results:
Weight 244
Miles: 3.01

TOF: 45 minutes, 01 seconds
14:58 average pace
546 cal

## I Hate Running: Unless It's Hell, Apparently.

If you hate running - like I do - you might like the Hell Run. Considering the name that seems like "liking" and "hell" is something you'd hear together only on "opposite day." Lemme esplain:

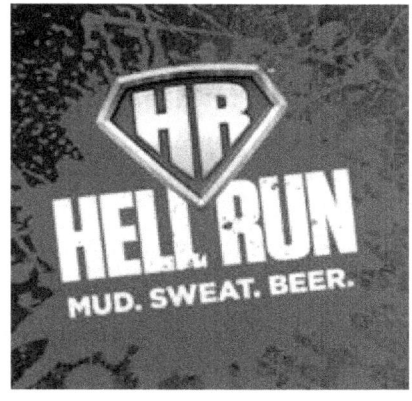

You already know that the droning thud-thud of my feet has had little interest for me since I was a wee lad. As the number of earth-sun-orbits I have experienced has increased, the joy of running has been replaced by an increasing hatred for this most primal of activities. Can't we evolve past this running thing, already? I have, however, enjoyed a few of the muddy adventure runs that I have experienced. This kinda freaks me out, because with a name like "Hell Run", you would think that mucking through watery slop, climbing walls, and crawling under barbed wire would mean LESS fun. You'd be wrong. Here's why:

## Obstacles

If running and climbing and ducking and slipping and falling and climbing and grunting sounds like fun to you, you are sick. While this does not sound like fun to me, IT IS. The obstacles remove the standard coma-inducing boredom that you normally experience while running, even providing you with something to look forward to. I know, it's *mortifying*. But it works. That primal satisfaction that real runner-types insist *is* a part of running actually works for me when I hit an obstacle. Is it the engagement of other muscle groups? Is it the satisfaction of climbing a 15-foot wall and overcoming an obstacle? Is it the satisfaction of stepping on someone's hand "accidentally" as you do so? I do not know. I do not care. It's fun. Dangit.

## Enthusiasm

Running sucks. As I said. MANY times. However, running around a bunch of other stupid/psychotic/crazy people has its advantages, and a general sense of group enthusiasm is one of them. If you are going to start a march for stupidity, you will probably be doing it with other stupid people. This is good as it makes you feel less stupid, or at least more content in your stupidity. This may be the greatest reason to enter ANY organized race, but muddy adventures like the Hell Run seem to be better at generating that kind of enthusiasm in its participants. This gives you an adrenaline boost that lasts for at LEAST the first 30 meters, if not a few more. So I guess It's like running a shorter race.

## Group fun

Running is typically a solo sport. Though our family runs together sometime, my wife's joy for running-as-meditation and my children's desire to zoom off on their scooters/humiliate the slow daddy has meant that even group runs are typically, well, not group runs.

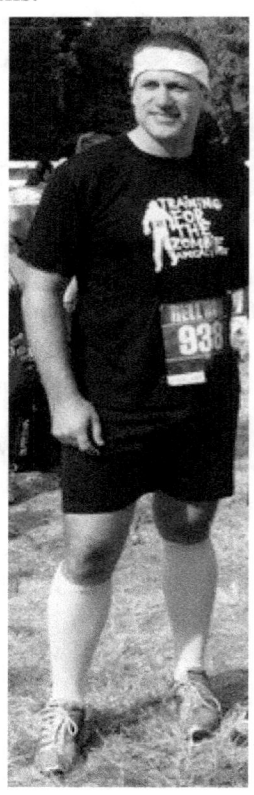

The Hell Run is different in that it's more of an "event", so we can share the experience with friends. We even play dress up a bit, which for me includes such radical moves as wearing a certain zombie training t-shirt, a bright green headband or neon socks. My friends this year took "dress up" even more seriously, wearing kilts, zombie makeup, or obnoxious you-can't-unsee-that tights.

## Beer

I am pretty critical of running, but is the return of my taste for beer a benefit? There is nothing quite like a nice cold brew after a hard run or workout or exercise regimen or bout of rigorous thinking or television show or nap.

We were outraged this year - outraged, I say - at another race we attended, the Warrior Dash, and their decision to allow Miller Light to be the sponsor and sole beer choice. You might be able to get away with that stuff in Arkansas, but in the Pac NW we like our microbrews and fancy IPAs. Hell Run was a total win with Alaskan Amber, and for this we thank you. Sherioushly. I love you, man.

## Music

Our Seattle Hell Run was treated to Tone Loc hisself this year, which was fun for us old fogies remembering the days when we meant something. It WAS a bit funny to see Tony Loc giving personal shout-outs to the three "brothers" in the crowd. That's not an exaggeration. While Seattle is a pretty liberal place, apparently this type of activity is still pretty homogenous in the type of folks it attracts. Sorry Tone. Still, us old white folks loved it.

Oh yeah, and don't forget there IS actual running.

This is what puts the "Hell" into Hell run. It's a short three miles, and except for the Hell/running part... it's a helluva lot of fun.

## 12. "THE MEASURE OF WHO WE ARE IS WHAT WE DO WITH WHAT WE HAVE." - VINCE LOMBARDI

I don't really read books on running very often. Scott Jurek's book is the exception. I have a book on lifting weights I got at Half-Price books. I have a guide to rock-hard abs. Other than that, my bookshelf is filled with books on business, the economy, motivational books, a few pieces of non-fiction, and science fiction.

What I'm saying is that I'm not a running afficianado. I'm not one of those annoying people that lives and breathes running. I'm not always training for my next race. All this talking about running is pretty new for me, let alone thinking about it. That's perfectly fine for other people, but I would more typically try to play something on the banjo, write something silly, or read an interesting article. Heck, I'd rather study statistics in my free time. I have done this. Creating the perfect body, or actually *working* on my health is a bit foreign to me, though I have had fun playing sports.

I want to enjoy running for its own sake. That's why yesterday's finish of my run by playing with my children felt like cheating. It's silly to feel that way. Of course it isn't cheating to run and play sports. I was, running, after all. When I ran as a child, it was because I was going somewhere. Why, then, do I feel like I need to enjoy running only in isolation?

And why should I think that running just to exercise *should* be fun? Is it possible that's the lazy man's way to think about it? Yes, it sure is. It's like saying I want results, but I don't want to have to put in the effort, and if it's effort I don't want to do it. I'd like rock-hard abs, I sure would, but those abs are going to have to come gift-wrapped and under the Christmas tree, or I don't want any part of it.

This is a very impatient, instant-gratification side of me.

I'm running near my house today. The Polar Vortex is coming, so it's a cool clear day. I wonder how we will talk about the "Polar Vortex" in 20 years. I bet we'll laugh at it, probably because it's a very scary term that basically means "we have cold weather coming." Calling it the "Polar Vortex" makes it sound like we're going to be whisked into another dimension, one based on Disney's Frozen. I sincerely hope that is not the case.

There's another alternative to why that term might be considered funny. We'll laugh about it because what those silly people around 2014 called a "Polar Vortex" is a ridiculously mild winter in 2034. But let's not think about that.

Anyway, it's cold. It froze last night. I can't complain with a spectacular clear sky, however. No hullaballoo about it, I just get out and go running. That's what runners do, right? They don't suit up, stretch for a half hour, warm-up, plan their route and get mentally prepared to run. They just lace up and take off. So I do.

My weight is holding strong at 244 pounds, so I've been meaning to have a pretty serious talk with myself about my diet. Diet and exercise are often mentioned together, I've heard.

Me: So listen, Self. I think you might be eating too much.

Self: Why do you say that?

Me: Because I'm running two to three miles a day and not losing any weight.

Self: Well maybe you need to run farther.

Me: Well that's a nice attitude. So now it's my fault.

Self: If the shoe fits...

Me: You don't have to change any of your own behaviors, right? You just keep eating what you want? Is that your solution?

Self: That's right.

(I don't think Self got Me's sarcasm)

Me: Good talk. Way to be a team player.

Self: Do we have any more pop-tarts at home? Oh, also, you're out of beer.

I notice suddenly that Me has a lot of sarcasm, but Self is very direct. Self gets what he wants, but Me is frustrated. There's a big lesson in here somewhere, but I'm missing it.

I'm running by an area of Mukilteo called "Possession Ridge." That's rather ironic, isn't it? First, possessing a ridge is a bit of a funny idea.

"See that ridge? I own it."

Second, running near the houses on possession ridge is an in-your-face acknowledgement of how money-grubbing we are, even in naming places. Tomorrow I'll run on Money street to ColdhardCash lane, which has an atm at the end of the street.

Still, I'd be lying if I said I didn't want to live on Possession Ridge. I'm sure it's a nice lifestyle.

I loop around the neighborhood streets. There are no sidewalks, but it's nice and sunny. It's hard to complain about being on a walk today, forget about running.

Cramping begins for me at about the fifteen minute mark. This is a concern because I've been blessedly cramp-free so far, and if cramping becomes a theme in my workouts, well, that is no Bueno.

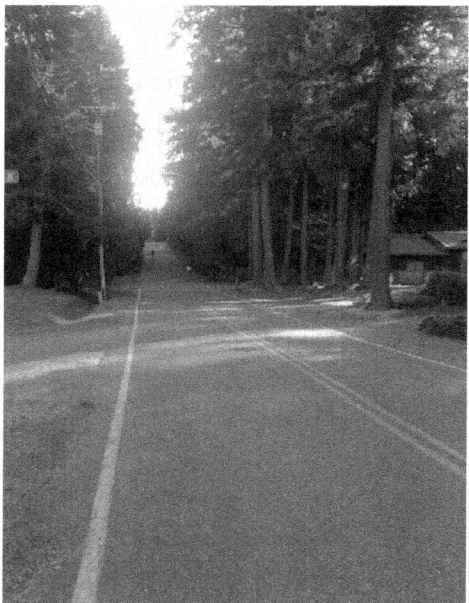

What I have enjoyed in this twelve-day period is mixing it up and running in different places. The Pacific Northwest is so beautiful. What's not to like about getting out in that? No matter what the consequences are, this whole experiment has been pretty worthwhile.

I find myself involuntarily slowing down, and thinking "This walking thing is kinda nice!"

Not a great run. I am surprised to look down at my watch and I'm already 28 minutes in. Is that a sign of increasing running capacity? I'd better hope it is. I will need that in a few weeks!

## Day Twelve Results: "Good effort"← thank you judgmental watch. Thanks. Is that sarcasm again?!

Weight 244
Miles: 2.63
TOF: 31 minutes, 10 seconds
11:51 average pace
471 cal
My mood: I want a twinkie.
My music reminds me as I end: "Keep Pushing. Keep Pushing." Thanks Steve Boyett.

## Gotta Be the Shoes

We have a Brooks outlet in Seattle and that's been my default shoe for years. I've worn Ravenna's, and we get them for around $30 at the outlet – not the latest model, of course. I've struggled with the Ravenna. I put Superfeet inserts in them, and they provide adequate support, but feel a little heavy and restrictive to me.

It was only recently that I discovered the Glycerin, and I love it. Even at my weight it feels lighter with adequate support. I don't use the Superfeet inserts. Now that's a good shoe for me.

On a related note, Nike shoes are, in my experience, excellent to look at. I mean, they really look great. Usually when I put them on I wonder why people would want to buy shoes that are physically painful to wear, but for some people looking good is just worth that sacrifice. If you want to look good for one or two runs before your feet turn into hamburger, then I would go with the Nikes.

I have a pair of toe-shoes, Vibrams, that I tried for a while. They are difficult to run in as they change they way you have to run. Some part of me thinks that isn't necessarily a bad thing – perhaps more of a back-to-nature style. I might go back to them sometime. I didn't get injured, and in fact found running in them a bit refreshing because it was so different.

I keep hearing lately about the Hokas, a ridiculous-looking shoe that some runners swear by. I am not too vain(only a little), so may end up giving those a try too someday. As we get a little older and more secure in our relationships, wearing a shoe that looks like a running clog isn't a deal breaker. In summary, if you don't mind not having sex for awhile or are in a secure committed relationship, you might want to give Hokas a try.

## 13. "GOOD AS IS DISCOURSE, SILENCE IS BETTER, AND SHAMES IT." – EMERSON

I hate Emerson. I discovered him in college, and he's almost unreadable. Not in a bad way. Yes, it's possible to be unreadable in a good way!

I actually am in awe of Emerson, which is the source of my hatred. Here's a guy who writes with thunderbolts, who practically claps his hands together, forms a sentence, and it's incredible. He's unreadable because every sentence is packed with import. It's inspired. It's like watching an Eddie Van Halen play guitar. He's so far ahead of anything you can do, you have so much respect, but also a tiny bit of hatred that every move by his fingers can seem magical, and it seems so effortless.

"Silence is better, and shames it." Ugh, that's classy. My inner monologue is shamed.

Emerson didn't write about running, to my knowledge. He did write about health:

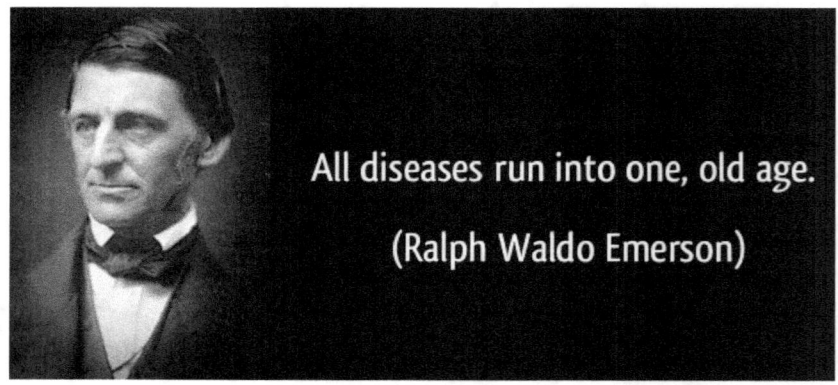

All diseases run into one, old age.

(Ralph Waldo Emerson)

Morning has broken in Washington, and it's a balmy 30 degrees outside. I take a cue from Emerson and run without music today. What will I do without my beloved music to run to? I have it on good authority that Emerson hated House music. I'm sure he never went to a Rave. I'm not even sure they had an equivalent in 1825. How did people party back then? An all-night revue of classical compositions? Yawn.

I have a phone interview today, which goes well. Of course, I always think it goes well. Hrm. But I eat a light lunch of a Peanut Butter and Honey sandwich and head out to the sunny frozen wasteland.

I'm running with my wife in the early afternoon. It froze last night, and as we start out we pass a frozen slug on the sidewalk. Sigh. A frozen slug! This is when your choice to get moving goes horribly wrong. That slug went out for exercise. He never came back. He sits on the sidewalk, a somber warning of what happens if you go out for a run when it is too cold.

See, I knew exercise was bad for you.

My wife doesn't think much of my slug commentary either. She takes off in front of me, so now I have to play catchup, dangit.

Running in silence is interesting. We get so attached to our gadgets. Every step we could be checking our watch for pace, or time or distance, or forwarding our song, listening to music the entire time, perhaps checking our heart rate monitor separately. Yeah, we run just like the cavemen did, with an iPod and pedometer, our fancy shoes and technical shirts. It's not a run, it's a fashion show. We run with more technology on our wrist than fostered in the industrial revolution.

It's another "meh" run. I force myself through a place where I feel like taking a walk break, twelve minutes in. A walk break is saying "I quit." The good running is right on the other side of that point, right beyond the place where you want to stop.

Day thirteen. Do I still hate it? I don't know. I'm ambivalent. After all, I'm only trying to change a few letters: from being an 'angry' runner to being an 'avid' runner. I'm trying to turn my experience as an angry, get in an argument with yourself, abjectly stupid, apish runner into being an "avid" runner. Just a few letters to change.

Can I do it? The jury is still out. I can see the allure of running, if I were a little more 'into' this. It's interesting to me when someone describes themselves as an 'avid' runner. That implies that they really enjoy it. Even the most seasoned runner will admit there are parts of it they hate, days that suck. When someone calls themselves an avid basketball fan, or an avid fisherman(fisherperson?), or an avid gamer, they don't secretly admit that there are parts of it they really hate. "Yeah, I like video games, but sometimes they are terrible." No, they're kinda not. Why is running different? Somehow, these people enjoy the process no matter the result. How is that possible with running? Seems more like running is a mental disorder, doesn't it?

As I near the halfway point near the library, I think about how this could be classified as a "good" run, but it's not particularly fast. There I go again, drawing a distinction between "running fast" and the possibility of having a good time doing it. Why is the idea of fun so dependent on being faster in my mind? Am I a closet running snob, and is my experiment doomed to failure because I can't overcome my own hangups about running?

## "You can never trust the human mind anyway. It's a death trap" – Anthony Hopkins

Maybe the purpose of this exercise isn't to fall back in love with running again. I mean, I have to be honest here. If I don't like something and I'm 46 years old, there's probably a reason. I'm older and wiser, right? Is the wizened me concluding that "this kind of sucks. You shouldn't do it." It may not be falling back in "Love" with running that I'm concerned with here. "Brainwashing" is more like it. Conditioning myself to enjoy the experience. Note to self: consider re-titling book "Re-Run: My 30-day Experiment to Hypnotize Myself to Love Running."

"Maybe," I tell myself sagely, "maybe I'm too smart for running. I have too many things going on in my head to get 'into' running. Running is for losers. I shouldn't like running, and if I do end up liking it, then I am effectively brainwashing myself."

That, ladies and gentlemen, is Tony overthinking this whole damn thing. I shake out the cobwebs of my thoughts. Don't overthink it. Just run. Anthony Hopkins also said: "We are dying from overthinking."

How can you experience something if you're always nattering to yourself about what you should be thinking or doing at any moment? You can't chase down clarity, you can't even enjoy something if you can't get outside your head. I'm like a baseball hitter that gets up to the plate and can't shake his thoughts enough to stay in the batter's box and has to call time before every pitch. I've got to get outside my own head.

That reference brought to you by the movie Bull Durham:

"Get a hit, Crash"

"Shut up."

Does this boil down to a nature versus nurture question? Are we wired for running, something we're born to, and is part of our natural state, or is it something we have to train ourselves to love?

Another running tip: It's helpful to run in front of someone of the opposite sex. Why? Because we're idiots. If you're running in front of a Chippendale dancer, or the Swedish bikini team, you run farther and faster to impress. You're not going to stop unless it's to throw up from exertion. You're not stopping until you get up around that corner there. We call that motivation.

Also, we call that Ego.

(Note to self: million dollar idea – The Bikini-model or Chippendale Dancer Half-Marathon. Okay, scratch that. You think that woman who walked through New York was accosted. These poor women and men might not finish the race. Needs: additional security.)

(Plus, very reliable sources tell me that running in G-strings is very uncomfortable and can result in painful chafing injuries to unlubricated parts.)

(Another note: if I do go forward with this, we might be able to sell tickets to the first aid tent. Or the Vaseline station.)

Walk breaks as usual today. I didn't exactly zoom back on my last half-mile. I'm not calling it fun. I'm just calling it a run.

## Day 13 Results:

Weight 242
Miles: 2.79
TOF: 30 minutes, 21 seconds
10:53 average pace
506 cal
My mood: get out of your head.

## 14. "THE SILENCE DEPRESSED ME. IT WASN'T THE SILENCE OF SILENCE. IT WAS MY OWN SILENCE."- SYLVIA PLATH

My story needs a protagonist. A young man who fights the forces of evil. Unwittingly, perhaps. Who doesn't know his own power, but grows in strength as he fights for the powers of good.

My story needs conflict, a challenge to be overcome. I will challenge and beat house Slytherin in Quidditch! Or discover my destiny through the tutelage of a diminutive troll doll who backwards talks he does.

Or I could break my leg. You know, just for the purposes of the story.

Well, that got morbid quickly.

I have officially run for a fortnight. I have never run consistently in my LIFE like this. I've run some 35 miles. That's 56k! That's worthy of celebrating, right?

So I've run a modem.

(You must be at least 30 years old to get that joke.)

Benjamin Franklin said "The problem with doing nothing is not knowing when you're finished."

So I'm doing something. Anything. I'm running every day in an attempt to rediscover what I used to love about it. I'm not sitting back on my duff waiting for inspiration. I'm creating it. There's value in that, no matter how much I grouse about it.

A running optimist might say: there are plenty of reasons NOT to run. You only need one reason to run.

A running pessimist might say: there are plenty of reasons to run. You only need one reason NOT to run.

A running realist might say: get your sorry ass out there and bicker with yourself later.

My story needs conflict? How about myself? How about the internal struggles of a guy pulling out all the stops to give running a try?

When I was young, we parted ways. I said goodbye to running because work took me away. I had other hopes and dreams. We grew apart. I fell in love with someone else. I even cheated on running with weightlifting. *Gasp!* The scandal!

So now I try to be faithful. It's my test. I run. I read blogs about running. I subscribe to runner's sites and feeds on twitter. I read books on running. I end up with an email about training for a marathon. Ha. Fools. Cool your jets, website autoreply.

I click on a link to "essential" gear a person needs to run, and it's all about being properly lit at night. People run at NIGHT? What strange hell have I descended into?

## Butterfly Effect

It's hard to think back on your life and imagine things you would change. I credit my skepticism of changing those decisions to science fiction. If I had made a different decision to buy a banana at a store, then through a series of circumstances I could have ended up a quadriplegic. Time travel is fickle like that. I like a lot of things in my life. I wouldn't want to have screwed that up by making a whole set of different decisions and rolling the dice.

I am thinking of this because I saw the movie Déjà vu with Denzel Washington last night. I had already seen it before, at least I felt like I had. You ever have that feeling?

But who doesn't like Denzel?! The movie was strangely unsatisfying, mostly because it answers one time travel question – can you change the past – spoiler alert, they do. It fails to answer the other time travel question – what happens when you do. That's really the big one. What would we have grown up as if we had changed some of our decisions as youth? Would you be a professional cricket player? An international Spy? Homeless?

(Have you ever noticed that if someone says "spoiler alert," it's too late to do anything? Like, "spoiler alert, he dies." WTF, man? We should give people a moment to cover their ears or something. Sorry about that.)

So live life without regret, is what I'm trying to say. Because according to time travel theories, you probably don't really regret even the worst of your decisions, because it will screw up your life and turn you into a butterfly. It's science.

Speaking of science, I have heard that science can help people run. It's probably an old wives' tale. So today I'm going to apply some fartleks as part of my run. I don't dare tell the children, or they will laugh for hours.

Fartlek means "speed play" in Swedish. So it's a game you play with yourself running distances. A fartlek is a short burst of energy, which I think has been abbreviated in English to just "Fart." That is to say, I'm going to go Fart it up out there today.

I think I just discovered the etymological root of Fart. Once again, committing yourself to a goal can pay unrealized dividends like this.

I'm feeling the fact that I'm only on day fourteen. I'm torn between being totally tired of this desperate attempt at self-relevance and paradoxically wanting to continue. Of course I choose to continue, mostly because if I stop now the book ends here. If you notice what page you're on, you know that doesn't happen. Spoiler alert.

Sometimes making a commitment to yourself isn't enough, but making it to others helps you stay motivated. And for this I thank you.

Motivation is that feeling of "aw, crap, I HAVE to do it now."

I have a phone interview today too. After I finish "wowing" the human resources folks on the phone(I'm sure that's what happened), I head out for my run.

I'm hitting Japanese Gulch again today(which, little known fact, was called "Jap gulch" at one point. Charming). I plan to run towards the water this time, which I have never done, down the train tracks. Hopefully it pops out somewhere near the water and I can make a nice loop around through the waterfront neighborhood in Mukilteo. Trying to mix it up, give myself a little different view. I'm running with music today because, forget Ralph Waldo Emerson. My silent head is scary and I want no part of that. I don't care how shameful it is. If silence is the truth, then I can't handle it. I'm going to go ahead and let my thoughts get permeated by the beat of sweet music and drown that stuff out. I know, shameful.

Fartleking is nothing more than a kind of interval training where you pick something out in the distance – a tree, a mailbox – and run toward it *faster* until you get to that point, where you slow back down. It can be super fast or reasonably fast, whatever. You can even incorporate walk breaks. So it's very much a way to work in intervals, but there isn't really a prescribed way to do it. It's loose, which appeals to me. I'm not a professional, ya know.

Oh, and forget about whether or not Fartleks are related to Farts in any way. That's debatable. But saying the word "Fartleks" does not sound right at all. Say it now. See what I mean? That isn't right.

If I can improve my running ability by getting in some fartleks today, well I'm all for it. I have noticed that when I run with the kids playing sports, I work different muscles. Hills have a different feel too, and Japanese Gulch is hilly. So if "running all out" for a period of time will help engage and develop different muscles and help me get stronger, I'm all for it. I do have that crazy half marathon at the end, so any little bit of toughness I can develop in the meantime is a huge benefit.

As I run down here, I realize I'm stacking the deck in my favor as a runner. I am setting this up as a nice beautiful downhill run, then uphill through a gorgeous section of Mukilteo. It's a bright clear day. After my bemoaning of the weather early this month, we've had some very good days. But I'm stacking the deck in my favor with this nice downhill run. It's going to be beautiful, I'll probably stop and take some pictures. A lot of good things in my favor, and the Fartleks should help me focus my effort on the course, which should keep me moving and help "gamify" the experience.

It's funny, I talk about running, and aspiring to fall in love with running. I follow Dean Karnazes on Twitter and check out running forums and blogs like "hungry runner girl" and "Running with Perseverance." These guys are so inspiring, but at the same time what they've done is so ridiculous. It's that feeling of "wow that's awesome!" followed by "OMG that guy is CRAZY." So here I am for 30 days proving I'm crazy too. Do I get to join the crazy club? I hope there is a patch I can sew on to things. Directly onto my skin.

It's very cold today, frozen temperatures still. I wind my way downhill as I step around and over frozen rivulets of water on the gravel trail. Exploring these parks is one of the best things about running. You get out in the great outdoors, see your own city or town. Mix it up if you do this, keep it fresh. Most cities have lots of city blocks. Why not run them all?

I turn down into the gulch and see a large train parked on the track. There is a sign a ways back up the track I've always wondered at. It says "do not walk within 15 feet of the tracks." That seemed like a lot to me, but now I see why. This train has large cargo containers, some stacked side by side on the railcar. They easily overhang six feet off the track. There's a trail down off to the left side that looks picturesque, so I take it.

It dives sharply down and crosses a stream twice – I can barely jump the distance. I take a picture of some very odd icicles on the grass nearby. It looks like they flash-froze. I'm pondering the embankment off to my left, which has risen to around 50 feet, and pondering how I'll get back up that way to where the residential neighborhood is. The trail winds its way up to the side of the train tracks again, on the far end of the train.

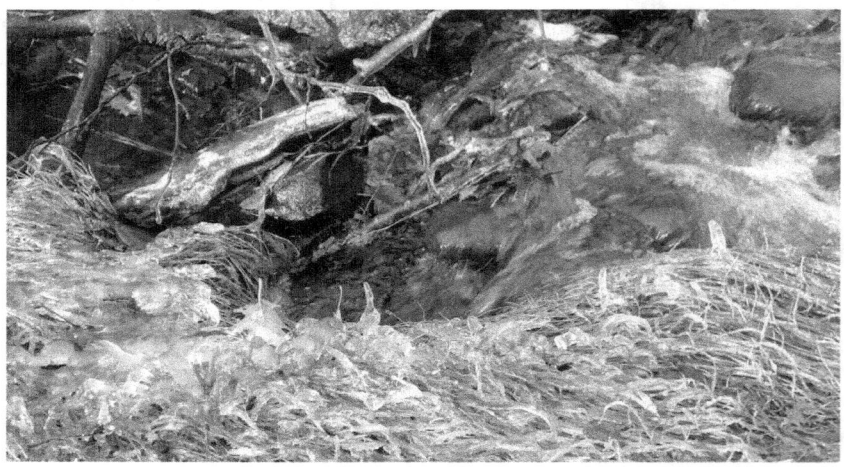

And then I see that I'll have to turn back, not five minutes into my run. It opens into the train track area, which has fences on both sides. I could run it, but I am not sure I can get out. So I turn around and jog back to the stream crossings, up the hill to the trailhead where I started. Oops.

I was always enamored with trains, not in a Sheldon Cooper(Big Bang Theory) kind of way, but in a "see the world" kind of way. As a youth, I imagined jumping a train car as it stopped and riding it to wherever it went. It's my hobo fantasy, and I don't think I ever shared that before. I would even dream up how I might survive a cold train ride on the outside of a train in freezing conditions. What to wear, how I might shelter myself, what to pack, what to eat. I didn't think there would be a nice empty railcar waiting for me; I thought it just as likely that I would have to hunker down on the top of a pretty full coal car, or on the back of one. A free and freeing way to move around, get off when I wanted, stay as long as I wanted. Leave.

Also, a pretty epic way to freeze to death.

I'm sure it's a Federal crime now, and what I just described would land me in what used to be called "the hoosegow." Ah, the times they are a changing sonny.

So rather than dwell on my upcoming visit to Joliet, I focus on the trail. Up the hill I go, fast as you please.

Okay, that lasted about twenty seconds.

Phew! I walk for a bit.

Fartleks. Gah. Whose dumb idea was it to do Fartleks up a danged hill. I quickly discover another peril of running in the Pacific Northwest: leaves in an otherwise clear forest looks suspiciously like a trail. That trail led nowhere, so I'm forced to backtrack. Again. Fartleks my ass. I'm trying to figure out where I'm going.

I figured Fartleks might play into my perceived strength: speed. Or at least the desire to go fast. But that really doesn't help when A) you're running uphill, and b) you have to keep backtracking. I keep going as best I can, running fast along the trail and slowing when I need to. It's my pace, after all.

I glance at my watch. Almost 20 minutes and only 1.2 miles. And I'm gasping for breath. What a wuss. C'mon Markey!

I apply the "what goes up must go down" principle and hit a good pace on my way back. I pass another runner going uphill, and wheeze out a lame "hello," which is only marginally better than raising my eyebrows at him as we pass(that's what he did).

Whatever frustration you have when you have to walk up a steep hill, you can take it all out on the downhill. I fly down.

I realize the serpentine nature of the trail, so my watch's distance might not be accurate. It's taking mini-snapshots of my location by satellite, and it isn't continuous, so it has to connect those snapshots into one run. That means a very windy trail may not reflect an accurate distance. Still, my pace makes me angry.

I know I'm pushing myself aerobically because this is just about as out-of-breath as I have been since I started. I can take some small consolation in that, but it feels a whole lot like celebrating suckage.

Unfortunately, due to my amazing time coming back downhill, I come back almost to the parking lot and have to jog left, back out another trail, to finish my time. I rock. Whine whine. First I moan about going too slow, now I'm saying I went too fast. Sheesh.

There DOES come a time in some runs where I "Feel it." During this run, that time is right now. I feel the energy in each footstep, and I bounce. I bounce to the music, I am being pushed along. There is an old running training exercise where you pretend there is a string attached to your breastbone, pulling you forward, as if someone is standing in front of you pulling it. Or is this an old acting exercise? Whatever. Go with it.

During these times you can throw your shoulders back, kick up your heels, and go at whatever pace you choose. Those moments are fleeting, and the moments you try to capture. But I do experience it, even if only for twenty seconds or so.

As I come back into the parking lot, I reflect on the fact that I thought I was stacking the deck with a nice loop, fartleks. None of that worked out. But I have no complaints. I felt it, I ran when I wanted to, I stopped when I wanted to. I should focus on that, forget about my whole pacing problem, just run when I want to run and walk when I want to walk. That alone might be enough to make me get better.

I'm right in my assessment as I look down at my watch to find out how far I went for this run. Ack.

## Day Fourteen Results:
Weight 242
Miles: 2.1
TOF: 30 minutes, 47 seconds
14:38 average pace
381 cal
My mood: Better. Almost inspired. ALMOST.

Honestly, the only reason that the accuracy of the distance is important to me is that I wanted to make a nice pretty graph at the end of the book. I wanted to look at my pacing and see if my pacing increased or my distance increased. For this run, since the watch didn't quite work properly, I will have to either leave this data point out or put an asterisk by it. It wasn't a bad run.

## 15. "GREAT THINGS ARE DONE BY A SERIES OF SMALL THINGS BROUGHT TOGETHER." - VAN GOGH

My friend and I drive to a bar. I sit in silence by myself – what am I doing, gathering my thoughts? –And then look to find him. He's angry at me now, for abandoning him as soon as we walked in. We sit together briefly, but he pointedly ignores me and watches TV, and then leaves to another room in the bar. I go after him when I realize he isn't coming back.

And it's a big dream-room bar with many rooms, so I flit from room to room, and everyone wants something from me, I am the center of attention. Hey, it's my dream after all. An older woman trips into me as I enter a room, she's a server, and she immediately starts dancing with me. I laugh and follow her lead, which is fun for a moment but gets uncomfortable. We part awkwardly, self-conscious.

Another room is mostly empty and I take a seat in a corner on some pillows. I'm looking at something, could be an iPad. And slowly people fill up around me, sitting just a little too close. Men and women. I have that feeling that people are aware of me, and somehow want to be around me. But I'm still looking for my friend, so I get up and everyone seems vaguely upset, like the party's over.

"We're on the fair board – do you want to be on the fair board?" A woman asks flirting. Yes, she asked "do you want to be on the fair board" in a flirty way. I say sorry, "I'm from out of town." I go through other rooms, which are really more "stores" than "rooms." One sells video games. One is a fast food joint. They are all interconnected, but none of them have my friend in them.

Dreams are strange vehicles into our subconscious. It was a noisy dream, full of distractions and frustration. I attract others and can't find my friend. It seems peaceful to wake to the world.

I awake to find my wife spoiling the children by watching "Project Runway" with our three boys. They love it. I suppress a scoff. First world problems.

But hey, it's Day fifteen I'm halfway through my running challenge!

I feel fitter, stronger, faster. But you know what? That attitude doesn't show up in the numbers. I'm not starting to kill it every run. I'm still running at about the same pace I started at. Can I run for longer periods? Perhaps, but it's not a dramatic increase. So while I feel better, that just may be my perception rather than the truth. Perception is reality, though, right? Feeling better about yourself is never a bad thing. Unless you're Jeffrey Dahmer. Then, you know, that's bad.

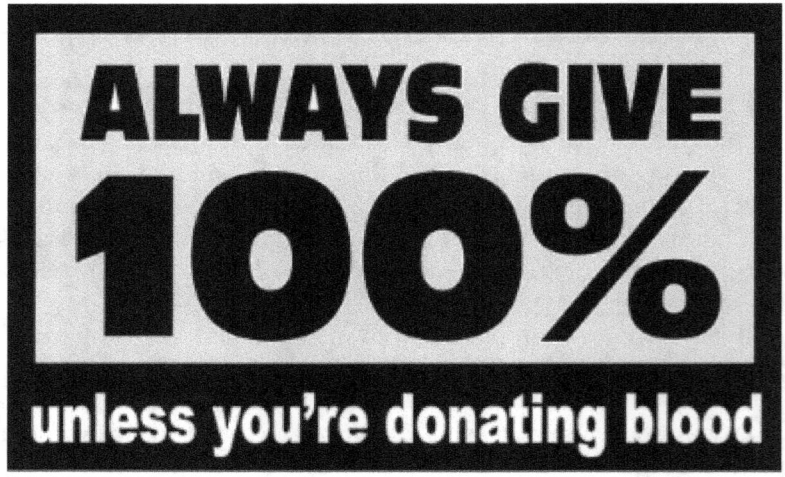

I'm back at Narbeck Wetland Sanctuary today for a FAMILY run. I am bringing all of my small things together, Van Gogh's advice. That means all three sons are here and my wife. We're all running together. It's a miracle I say.

Our middle son, Aidan, runs cross-country, and while he enjoys it and has fun, inspiring him to greater heights has been a challenge. Whenever we urge him to run outside of cross-country, he shrugs and agrees he should, but never wants to run. So getting him and the whole family out here today seems like it's time for a hallelujah breakdown.

Everyone else takes off, but my watch refuses to sync because I don't know, solar flares probably. Smog in China. And me without my tinfoil hat. So I leave the parking lot later than everyone else, hoping to catch them. Oh, who am I kidding. I shouldn't disillusion myself like that. I'll never catch them.

It's another nice clear, cool day, so I am totally lucking out with the weather this November. I feel good – happy to be halfway through, that's for danged sure. The excitement I feel, strangely, translates into the feeling of "I am interested in going running today."

Do any of you real runners play this game with your watch where you wait for the watch to sync up, hold your arm up to the sky – like you are a rabbit-ear antenna and holding your hand 24 inches closer to the satellite will solve the problem? It doesn't. And then you hold perfectly still, like that has been the problem all along: the satellite can't find you. Does that work? Or are we all just being morons? Or…. Is it just me being a moron.

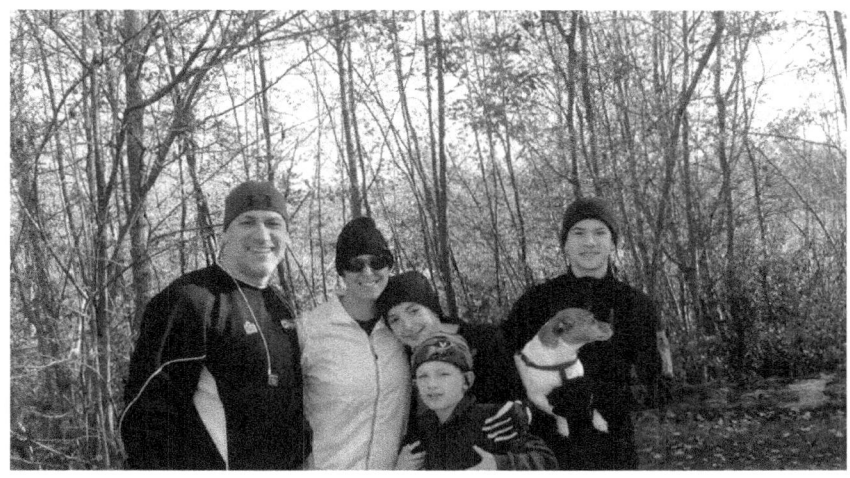

Here's my danged cute family, along with their patriarch(that's the one standing next to the Matriarch).

I take off into the frosty forest. My watch never syncs up, so about a quarter of the way through my first lap I hit the stopwatch.

I kick through leaves along the trail. My children have annihilated my time, which I'm sure they don't realize. That wasn't their intention, to humiliate their father with their youth and natural speed. And yet here we are. Them: bounding ahead. Me: futilely flailing behind.

Always encouraging to see some work being done in the park. A couple new patches of gravel placed out there, where there were only puddles last time. Nice job gang.

As I complete the first lap, about 1.1 miles, my wife comes out of the interpretive trail section and slides in behind me. Well, great. Now I HAVE to run fast. So of course, what do I do? I don't stop. That would wound my ego.

And of course I stop a few minutes later. I come to a realization. I was never as fast in my youth as I thought I was. All of my speed was optimism, the exuberance of youth. Belief may have colored my reality.

When I was in the Seventh grade I challenged my stepfather to a footrace near our house in Fairbanks, Alaska. I was faster than him, I knew it. I mean he was OLD. And I was young. It was an impromptu thing, just a 100 yard dash or so thing near our house.

Honestly, I never thought of losing. Running was a part of me. Running was who I was. I ran all the time. He was just an old guy that did construction that married my mom.

Oh, did I mention he was pretty physically fit, and half native-American? Did I mention that part?

Well, the story ends but not exactly surprisingly. He did what every red-blooded American male would do and whupped my ASS. I had him for the first seven or eight centimeters, but when we got to actual meters, it was never a close race. Whoosh. And Whoops.

Later, my stepdad would race someone else around the "pond", a man-made lake that float planes landed on in Fairbanks, Alaska. The course was probably two or three miles. He beat them too. Small consolation for me. I never considered that our initial race might have been the inspiration for his race later, but I'm sure that's true.

So see, I was such an amazing runner I inspired other people to run. (If you spin it right, your resume can still reflect success in the midst of failure, right?)

To be fair, I wasn't slow. But in the grand scheme of things I was probably just a little better than average. There's no delusion of speed in my present self; but I can't shake the delusions of youth. I can't shake that competitiveness, which exists for no other reason than to gratify my ego.

Running is a solitary sport. As it turns out, I am woefully underprepared for it.

I run faster to catch my wife. She passed me, but I try to catch her. I surge ahead. She's nowhere to be seen.

"I married a robot," I think.

She's got some wind, that girl. That's what happens when you get serious about running. She ran thirteen half-marathons in 2013. THIRTEEN! One every month, a bit more. Talk about impressive. Again, very inspirational. My wife is a self-made runner, too. She was fast in school, but she never ran track, so she had to work for everything she's got. In the process, she dropped 80 pounds. Very much a running success story. I guarantee you that without her effort and example I would not be out here right now. I would not be here, sucking wind, gasping for breath. Thanks honey. *Gasp*

I come out onto the street part of the trail, and find out that my wife has taken a left out of the trail instead of a right. She's going for more distance today. Showoff.

Superstar. Awesome. Freakish showoff.

Lap two means I pass the children again, bounding along. Like rabbits. Running through the fall leaves. If you want to get inspired to go running, watch the joy on their faces.

I meet my wife on a lap of the interpretive trail.

"How are you enjoying the interpretive dance portion of the trail? Have you already used all your best dance moves?"

"Yep."

"What do you call your performance pieces?"

"huffing and a chugging."

I jog with her through the interpretive trail, about a quarter mile.

Someone came up with the idea that you need 21 days to develop a habit. That sounds like an oddly specific number. Why not twenty days, or 22 days and eight hours?

I can tell you this: running for fifteen days in a row has given me the expectation that I will go running. I wake up every morning, not worried and thinking "ugh, I have to run today," but more like thinking "I am going to run today." That's something. Creating the habit is something great for my own physical fitness. I can't say I am totally looking forward to running every day, but the expectation is something. Perhaps the magic twenty-one days will seal the deal and I'll be a runner forever, an irreversible transformation into Meb Keflezighi.

Today: the kids had a great time. The dog had a great time. I involved my family and I have not a single complaint about how the run went. I continue to run, making incremental steps(literally) forward toward my goal of running for 30 days. Come what may, that's a major victory.

## Day 15 Results

Weight 241
Miles: 2.74 (mapmyrun)
TOF: 34 minutes, 00 seconds
12:24 average pace
Mood: I'm feeling good! How are you?

## "Oontz Oontz Oontz"

Music is a generally inspiring thing when running. I put on Steve Boyett's *podrunner* episodes when I run, which has saved more runs than

I can count from total boredom and/or a suicidal depression spiral. So I guess I owe you my life, Steve.

(Tony Markey accepted no compensation for this endorsement. I only know the man by his work.)

I can't tell you how much listening to music helps me. It makes me feel, like the time is flying by, and I am too. Anything with a beat helps. I try not to think about how this is obliterates silence. I don't like silence, if you haven't figured that out. I do like house music, the rhythmic nature of it, and I think it lends itself to running with the right tempo.

## 16. "WE DON'T SEE THINGS AS THEY ARE. WE SEE THEM AS WE ARE." - ANAÏS NIN

There is nothing better than hanging out with friends.

Last night we went over to our neighbor's house and they had another couple over, another neighbor. It's wonderful to have discourse with people, which was wide ranging, from being an Iranian in Alabama, to Armadillos in Oklahoma. Living in Italy. Visiting Amsterdam's Red Light District. Ironically, almost none of the stories were about traveling.

Have you ever noticed that stories of traveling are never about traveling? They are about what happens, what interesting experiences we had, and invariably the experiences aren't "quintessentially" that nationality. We don't tell tales of hour our experience in Mexico was so very Mexican, and doesn't that experience capture the spirit of Mexico and its people so well. Humans around the world are remarkably alike, at the end of the day. Our stories are our perceptions of the world, nothing more, and those are little more than musings on a situation, colored by our perception. Traveling without leads to traveling within, and suddenly we have stories about being in a hot tub in Canada which could easily have happened in the United States only it didn't, because we had to travel somewhere to laugh in a hot tub.

Our host, a bright physician from Italy, told the story of buying a birthday cake in Minnesota. The cake-selling clerk hadn't made "nature's leap," as he called it in his thick Italian accent. For those of us who also haven't made nature's leap, I think he meant she was dumb. He asked what kind of cake it was. "Chocolate," she said. The cake was covered in brown frosting, so he figured it was chocolate frosting, but he wanted to know what was inside. "I understand that," he replied, "but what kind of cake is it?"

"It's an *American* cake," she responded. Obviously she had guessed at this point that her customer wasn't from Minnesota, and was doing her best to start over with a more basic understanding of what a cake meant. In *America.*

Our host described the rest of the interchange, where he asked her what kind again because he wanted to make sure that it didn't have "juices" in it, and she repeated *"American"* and *"Chocolate"* over and over. Slowly.

As he told it, it was obvious that the clerk meant that the inside of the cake was chocolate in addition to the frosting being chocolate, but he didn't really get that, even years later. Their dialogue had turned into a comic memory.

Years later, he regaled his guests with tales of a dumb cake lady.

Years later, she probably tells her dinner guests of the dumbest customer she ever had.

Our memories are tinted by our perceptions and assumptions. I'm running to find out what is inside the cake. What flavor is running, really? Is it delicious? And I have to ask myself, am I the dumb clerk or the dumb customer?

My eldest son is a wonderful guitar player, a trombone player, a great student, he plays soccer and basketball, acts in school plays, has been on student council... Yeah, he's that guy, just an all-around superstar. I brought him down to Redmond today to play music with his group at church. While he plays, I'm going to go running on the Sammamish River Trail, arguably one of the best places to run in the Seattle area. I park just south of Woodinville to get onto it. The Sammamish River Trail is where runners go to run. It's always densely populated with runners, bikers, and walkers. It's a serious training area. I feel like a serious runner as I put my stocking cap on near the baseball fields and head to the paved bike trail near, which parallels the river all the way into Redmond.

I start with a little Banjo music. Some Jalapeno Flashback with Jeff Scroggins. Bluegrass has the wrong cadence for me to run to, but the banjo has always made me happy. The good stuff has incredible drive and gets me going. Someone described the sound of a banjo as firecrackers in a bathtub.

Uh, no offense bikers. I know you are doing something, you're getting out there, and that is fantastic, but why are there so many overweight bikers fitting their 250 pound frame on a tiny bike? It's like going to the gym and walking by the Zumba class. You don't often see the thin people in Zumba. It's great to get out there, but if you're getting out there week after week and you still weigh the same IT'S NOT

WORKING. If you're out there to have fun, that's absolutely good. But if it's a weight loss thing? Reconsider.

Look at me, the shining example. I haven't lost a single pound. Nary a pound. Zilch. I'm such a shining example. So STFU, self. IT'S NOT WORKING.

Frozen and clear again today. The Sammamish River is even more popular with wildlife than with people. Some kind of egret flies overhead at my starting point, dark grey with an orange bill. They fly away if you get near them in the wild, but this one just gives me a wary look as it passes twenty feet over my head. Gorgeous.

Bikes flash by me at 800 miles per hour. A couple people run by me as well, really fast. A fifty year old guy that might as well be riding a bike, holy smokes. I'm thinking "do I qualify to be out here?"

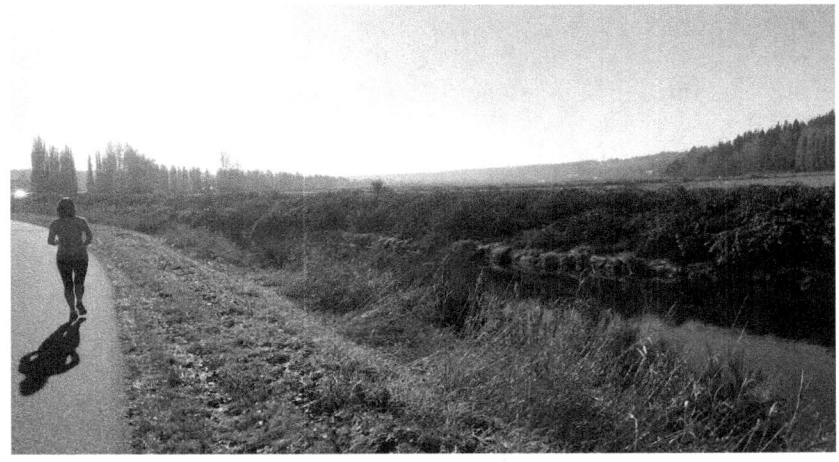

I wave and smile to people as I go by. It's amazing how few people interact on the trail. Of course this is near Redmond. I've met some stuckity-up folks from this area. Maybe it's the location. I've always tried to acknowledge other people as I run; after all, we're all out here trying to do the same thing!

As I roll along between the poplar trees and the river, I'm thinking how fortunate I have been with injuries. No twisted ankles, significant soreness, shin splints, very little cramping, and not even blisters. It's as if my body has been *waiting* for me to challenge it. Isn't that a healthy way to think about it? Your body is waiting for you to challenge it. Despite my initial concerns, whether I believe it or not, in a very real way I am already a runner. I have a body that's fit enough to drag my sorry butt out here for two or three miles every day. Doesn't that make me a runner already? Have I been in denial my whole life about this?

Am I just negotiating the flavor of the frosting? Have I always been a runner on the inside?

What I'm saying, with all due humility, is that my body's all cake. In my Ryan Gosling voice: "Hey girl, want some cake?"

Author's note: I don't have a Ryan Gosling voice. I used to do a passable impression of Danny DeVito. Will that suffice?

It's comfortable in the sun, but when you dip into the shadows of the trees it quickly drops below 40 again.

## The flavor of the cake is Nichtwissen

I'm coming to another significant conclusion: my greatest obstacle is my head. It's the biggest impediment to my running. I'm thinking about running wrong, probably for most of my life. I can't even trust my own perceptions of "like" and "dislike" because I've been thinking about dislike and running in the same context for so long, I don't know if that's really the way I feel or not.

There's a term for this feeling; it's the german word "nichtwissen," which means a consciously perceived lack of knowledge. I know what I don't know. Worse, I don't know whether or not I can know it. I perceive that I don't know what I don't know, and may never know.

In my mind, I'm both the seller of the cake and the buyer, and neither party knows what type of cake it is, but the argument continues.

It's the ultimate doubt. It's the acknowledgement of how stupid we really are.

Plutarch said "What we achieve inwardly will change outer reality," and this is what I'm feeling on day sixteen: that it's as if I am starting over. My mind, over a period of years, has been playing tricks with me regarding what running means, what it represents, and whether or not I "am" a runner.

THIS is the real purpose of my experiment, to get back to my own truth. It's not important to get faster. It's not important of focus on time, pace, distance. It's just as important to focus on the one, the *only* thing: running.

Even the one parameter I've set for myself: a total time of 30 minutes a day, skews my perception and leads me astray. I find myself focusing on the time because I might be close to my goal rather than experiencing the "goal" of running for its own sake. You've probably noticed that my times are always around 30 minutes? That is the goal I have set for myself, so I take pride that I am achieving it – but I don't go much farther. Why is that? It might be because I'm focusing on the wrong things.

I have always focused on the wrong things.

The idea of running is to lose yourself, and if you set these artificial parameters around doing your best, beating someone, competitive this and personal record that, you may be setting yourself up for failure before you begin.

There have been great benefits for me already as part of this experiment, in terms of motivation, in terms of keeping what amounts to a kind of diary and logging my thoughts, and having solitude. Instead of focusing on the details, I just need to go out and run and see how I do, and then go out and run the next day and see how I do. As it sits, I am putting such a microscope on everything that it is difficult to relax and enjoy the experience – which is entirely the point.

I'm at the turnaround point now. I resolve to let the music play, let the drummer kick, put the pedal down and enjoy myself on the return leg back to the car.

The good news! The start of the last two weeks seems like I am being pulled to the finish line already. I feel an inescapable conclusion I am being drawn towards, some inexorable gravitational well to the center of the truth. I really don't know what that is yet. It's a black hole, sucking me in.

Sylvia Plath be damned. Sometimes my own silence is okay. And I'm a damnably interesting person. "I'm good enough, I'm smart enough, and doggone it, people like me."

It's the end of the run, so I'm having my motivational moments. I use this impetus to drive me a little faster. A group of mallards coast into the water next to me. I'm way over time today, but it's nothing a hot bath can't fix.

Have you had a near-death experience? I have, and it sucked. A medical condition took me to a place where I can say I'm pretty fortunate to be above ground, let alone in possession of(most) of my faculties. I know I haven't shared that until today, but it suddenly seemed important.

My wife posted a wonderful article about near-death experiences recently – how we expect those who have had a brush with death to be different, unfairly so. We expect all of their crap to disappear. I am proud to announce that I am the same messed up jackwad I was before that experience. Isn't that wonderful? Being almost dead doesn't have to change you into anything more than you were before – you can take your baggage with you, wherever you go!

In today's world of problems, we should be grateful for whatever we have. There are dark times in our lives, and this challenge is helping me work through some of those thoughts. Sometimes we wonder why we live in a world that is this way, that has *insert world problem here*. Climate change, terrorism, a comet smashing into us, Ebola, an ineffective congress, the staggering number of cat videos on the internet, all these things make us unsure of where the world is going.

Sometimes it's enough to be alive.

I finish this run with a thought that's only cheerful if you've had a near-death experience:

"Just remember, your day could be worse -
You could be dead."

## Day 16 Results:

Weight: 243
Miles: 3.16
TOF: 39 minutes, 01 seconds
12:17 average pace
577 kcal
Mood: Nichtwissen

## 17. "WE MUST MAKE THE GOAL CONFORM TO THE INDIVIDUAL, RATHER THAN MAKE THE INDIVIDUAL CONFORM TO THE GOAL." - HUNTER S. THOMPSON

I am a wolf that hunts and eats. The wolf goes to sleep content and wakes up hungry.

Not hungry for running. If you read that as I am "hungry for running" you totally read that wrong. Ha, no way. <wipes tear> No.

Each day, I go to bed excited that I'm making progress towards my goal. I really do. I gain a sense of strength and speed throughout the day as I accomplish what I set out to do. Then I wake up the next day, wary that I have so much more to do. It's a good way to live, isn't it? Like every day is a march to a happy ending. What happens if I keep feeding the wolf?

I plan a short trip to Langus Riverfront Park in Everett today, just north of the city of Everett, a trail that borders the Snohomish River as it flows to meet Puget Sound. They shake hands. It's all very friendly. It's another estuary, so I imagine I'll see a lot of waterfowl today also. That never gets old.

Something else I'm experiencing in my life right now: sometimes you advance yourself in little ways, through civic meetings and participation, through a letter to the editor of your hometown paper and a few comments to a soccer coach or PTA president. It's truly amazing what a difference you can make just advancing a few thoughts with people. Advocating for yourself. People might even take you seriously. This is incredibly gratifying, being involved in a very real, human way in your little piece of the world. This also has the effect of giving you strength in other things. Often, you don't have to be smart, funny, urbane, sophisticated. Of course I am all of these things, I know because I chant that to myself every night before I close myself.

I'm just saying you just participate, and your contribution is important. Again, an upwards spiral of self-confidence and power.

"You may be keeping accounts, and presently you shall walk out of the door that has seemed to you the barrier of your ideals, and shall find yourself before an audience – the pen still behind your ears, the ink stains on your fingers – and then and there shall pour out the torrent of your inspiration." Stanton Kirkham Davis

I did a show in graduate school called "The Actor's Nightmare" by Christopher Durang. In it, an actor quite literally ends up on stage with no idea what he is supposed to do or say. Nonplussed. A nightmare, truly. A comic moment, to be sure. But running is shrugging this off of me as I make incremental progress towards something. The way I'm feeling, even in reflective moments, is a bit exhilarated. I have to admit, that could be addictive.

Is running Oxycontin for the soul?

Okay, that suddenly doesn't sound so great.

It's not the same thing as developing a love for running, in and of itself, though, is it? I am reminded of the old adage that no one wants to go to the hardware store and buy a drill. Rather, they want a hole in something. No one wants to run. They DO, however, want the results of running.

Ergo, all people who say they love running are liars, right? Must be.

It's a working theory.

Langus Riverfront Park is a bit off the beaten path for me, and it continues my grand tour of the parks and trails within about 20 minutes of my house. Again with the cool, clear days. Gorgeous. It's still November, right? What the heck.

You can see the mountains beckoning off in the distance, two of them are covered in snow already. This weather is my favorite to run in. Running in the rain is inspirational in a "no-one-else-is-dumb-enough-to-do-this" way, but when it's cold and clear your body warms up while running, and the cold helps regulate your body temperature. The air has that nice fall crispness. Hey, if I don't like running after this, you can't blame nature.

I would like to announce that due to careful thought, due to my and resolve of purpose, and with all due magnanimity, I will not be running with my watch today. I would like to announce that I have decided that watches are for wimps and I will no longer be tied to the technological crutches that prevent us from achieving our true communion with nature.

I would like to say to all you watch wearers: "Free yourself of this vile instrument of evil, from the cruel despotism of technology!"

I would like to announce that, but it's really not true. I just forgot my blasted watch today.

I feel naked without my watch.

Will my stopwatch work? It's on my phone. It's sensitive, I might have turned it off again as I put in in my little fashionable fanny pack that I wear.

I say "fashionable." There's no such thing. My fanny pack is unobtrusive, being little more than a waistband with a small pouch in it. I wear it under my shirt when I run. Men: why can't we get a man-purse handled? This would be a valuable thing, but we can't seem to make such a thing socially unacceptable. Go look to Zach Galifinakis for inspiration on the internet. That's an inspiring image, isn't it?

Anyway, stopwatch, of course that's bugging me now. We're so tied to gadgets, all of them. All of them are pointless when you're just trying to run.

An egret takes off near me. Birds are everywhere. I'll have to take pictures today.

This entire trail circles around the Snohomish River, looping back and forth through the wetlands and over streams. It's incredibly peaceful. Let's see if I can experience some of that peace running today.

I'm jolted out my running reverie by something unexpectedly disgusting. Coffee burps. Hoo. Yuck. I'll have to reconsider coffee I think.

And that was the moment I gave up on my challenge!

Some dredging is happening in the river today. They are probably looking for someone who had coffee burps and decided to end it all? I nod grimly. I get it fella, it's awful.

Anyway, peace. I'm focusing on peace now. This park is peaceful. A great place to see waterfowl. As a result, there are always people here with cameras.

I stop to take pictures. My stopwatch isn't working, I note. #wecanlandonacometbutwecant make a stopwatch on a phone that won't stop accidentally. That gag for you twitter users. #firstworldproblems #ihatehastags.

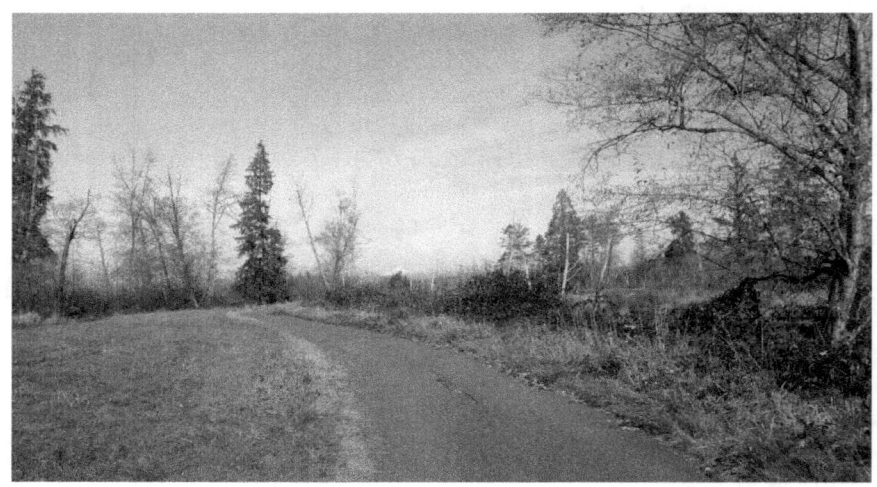

I see a hawk in flight. He's scanning the landscape for delicious woodland creatures. Moles, voles. I'm just assuming rodents because there are no "Hawk-o Bell" or "Jack in the Hawk" restaurants nearby.

I'm just communing with nature, man.

I jog across the metal-and-wood bridge to Spencer Island. It looks like an abandoned scene, one where you might film a zombie movie. I'm not sure why I'm so fascinated with zombie films, because sometimes they are terrible. Okay, they are almost always terrible. And they always have too much gore. Many of them are unwatchable. I can almost count what I consider the really good zombie movies on one hand. It's an underdeveloped genre – but thankfully that's changing.

I don't even like horror films, but I enjoy zombie movies and particularly the series The Walking Dead and even a lesser-known(and not quite as good) series called Z Nation. So what's the attraction?

I think it's the pseudo-survivalist in me, the person that knows that nature holds many secrets, the Alaskan that loves hearing stories for whom modern life is reduced to a shambles. They have to get back to nature, to their roots. That's the real exploration in those movies. They are stories human survival in a world they knew well, but which has become violent and in some ways unrecognizable. That's the interesting part. Out here, running in nature, it is the same kind of struggle. Man against himself, ultimately.

We came here earlier in the summer with the kids, but now part of the trail we took is under a few feet of water. That part of the trail heads straight out into the wetlands. So I run to the right, on what I think is a small loop. The only problem with running this park is that its beauty is distracting. It's a spectacular day and the perfect time of year, as it turns out. I turn off my music(you do WHAT?!). Yeah, it's that amazing. I actually want to go farther out on my run today.

As you run across the trail and over a bridge through the wetland, you have a 360 degree view of the park and the teeming wildlife.

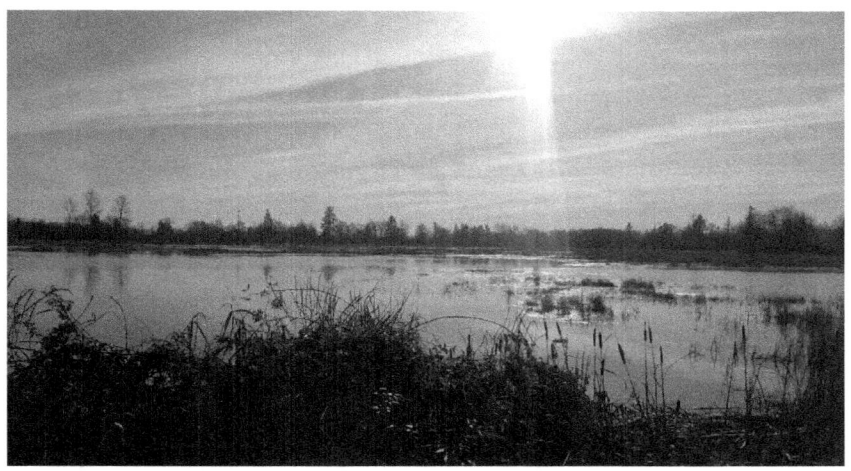

I keep ambling along, and pass a man that looks so comfortable in the park he looks like he might just have walked here from his log cabin on the other end. Some people are very comfortable in nature – and not nearly as comfortable with people. That describes practically everyone I knew in Alaska. I've met them in Montana, Idaho, and Washington too. I am a "greenhorn," and proud of it. Someone not so comfortable out of doors. I believe that we invented fire and houses for a reason, and I intend to use them whenever I can for their rightful purpose.

"Hiking?" I used to tell people, "In Alaska we just called it going outside."

In the Eleventh grade we lived in a house that had no running water. No electricity. The walls were unfinished plastic sheeting with insulation underneath. My first job when I came home was to build a fire. I did homework many night by the light of our propane lanterns(when we had propane), or by candlelight.

So I'm not really that big on camping. Some part of me feels I've camped puh-lenty, and I really like warmth and heat. I really really do.

I've stumbled into a run longer than 30 minutes, but it's so danged pretty. I'll take this path and hope it connects. A red hawk circles above me.

He's up there gliding, laughing at me. I would, if I could fly. Wouldn't you look down and say "what kind of stupid way of getting around is using your *legs*?" and "you call yourself an evolved species?" Yes, I would totally heckle people.

At this point I'm not sure how far I'm running anymore. I think I read that there is a seven mile loop here somewhere. So if I accidentally took that loop, please tell my wife and kids that I love them after they discover my body.

This is a true trail run, a nice wide path but bumpy, as if it was carved from nature or something. I have to concentrate on my footfalls, but I'm actually having a lot of fun. Running, walking, enjoying it. Immensely. From a technical running perspective, this may be the most fun I've had. Running through the marshes, focusing on where my feet go, and so much to see. The essence of running, is, of course, play. How could I grow up to not like play?

I come around the corner of the trail and see the end, where I'm connecting back to. I involuntarily say "hurray!" and scare the heck out of a flock of ducks. They take off, quacking angrily, creating a large rush of water as they put distance between us. Well excuuuuuse me.

I've seen countless ducks, a heron sitting on a stump, an eagle… oh, and now I hear gunfire off in the distance. The northern part of this estuary has an area for hunting. So I won't stray up that-a-way. Well, I hope they shot dinner.

I cross a bridge and startle a hooded merganser, a beautiful bird. He was paddling quietly, saw me, and freaked out. Quaaaaack!!!!!

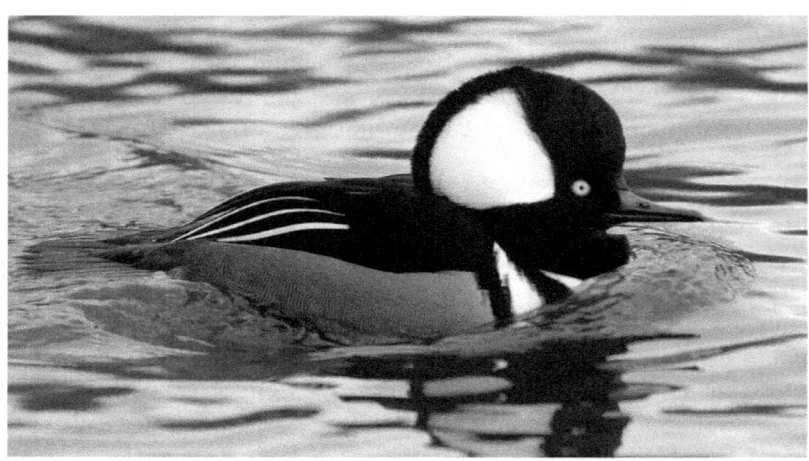

Don't worry buddy, didn't you see the signs? I can't shoot you on this part of the park! He doesn't listen.

Some folks have a habit of leaving their dog's poop bundles by the side of the trail. That. Is. HILARIOUS. It's as if that dog owner said:

"My dog pooped, and I couldn't just leave it there. So I thought I would wrap it up nicely and leave it for you. Merry Christmas."

I thought that the parks I had run through so far on this challenge were amazing, but this is inspirational. Either that or I'm turning into some kind of hippie running freak. This summer with the family it was very dry and hot, with little to see. Autumn on Spencer Island is a haven for wildlife. An absolute treasure.

Just a wonderful day and a fun(gasp!) run.

I stop by Burger King on my way home. I can't think of a hawk pun to go with that. I should have stopped at "Jack in the Hawk," but I needed some kind of bad pun closure here. I got nothing. Don't think less of me.

## Day 17 Results:

Weight: 243
Miles: 4.00(mapquest)
TOF: 50 minutes, 00 seconds(estimated)
12:50 average pace(est)
Mood: Fabulous

## Stop the bleeding

You know those friends with all the over-the-top crazy problems in their life?

Stop bleeding on yourself, people. Don't we all know people who always seem to have insanely difficult problems? These are the ones that get on Facebook and "vaguebook" about them, like "Worst. Day. Ever." Or "I can't stop crying…" ← an actual post. News flash. They are not insanely difficult problems. They are not unique, never-before-seen problems of humanity. To be sure, they might be terrible. But vaguely venting about them on social media only creates drama. What's the point of that nonsense?

They bleed on themselves. They are always lactating. They always sacrifice so much, and you should really listen to them. They are the proverbial Jewish grandmothers. The important thing is not the sacrifice, but that everyone around them is aware of their sacrifice. Their pain. Who cares about your sacrifice. Did Ghandi worry about his sacrifices? No, he died, you self-aggrandizing twit.

Anyway, we all have problems, and yes, some of us have bigger problems some of the time. News flash: no one cares about our problems. If you find that your problems trump the people you know almost every time, then I would suggest that:

You don't know their problems as well as you think you do, or
Yours aren't as big as you think they are.

"People only like conversation because they get to talk next," someone said. We all want to talk. How refreshing it is for those who listen!

Work your stuff out.

# 18. "THE MAN ON TOP OF THE MOUNTAIN DIDN'T FALL THERE." – VINCE LOMBARDI

Morning has broken, and I head outside to chop down some blackberries in our yard. Not the delicious fruit, but the gnarled, thorny branches that produce them. Blackberries are notoriously invasive, and every year it's man versus nature in our struggle to beat them back before they get too established as they creep towards our yard from the nearby native growth area. The blackberry bushes are so thick, I have to cut each of them into foot-long pieces so the intertwined branches start to separate. And each running branch is more than ten feet long. How can something so delicious be so annoying?

I have the same thoughts about running. The end result of running, being more physically fit, is desirable, but how to deal with the thorny middle? Do I have to let the idea of loving running invade my soul to be able to tolerate it long enough to get to the fruit at the end of the season? Am I mixing metaphors?

At the end of the day, does it matter if I like everything ELSE about running except the actual running? At a certain point, isn't it "all good?" Or am I the petulant child who will not eat his green beans, no sir, and will pick around everything on his plate so I don't have to eat any green beans? I want the benefits of health, but am I simply too dumb to know that there is work involved – and there always will be?

I actually worry about someone picking up this book(say, you, for instance), and getting all inspired and crap like that and going out and trying to run a few miles, and it's too hard for them(you). I worry that for some reason, my experiment seems like the culmination of a lot of ideas in my life, and I'm succeeding in it despite my past failures. But maybe someone(you) has had a few more shakes than I have, or drinks a bit more beer, or has played a lot more video games(how is THAT possible?). Maybe you can barely walk a mile.

Or maybe you're like some people and you run like a damned gazelle and you're sick of all my ridiculous whining, well maybe then screw you pal.

Sorry, Sorry, I got a little ragey there. My humblest of apologies.

My point is that we each have our own journey. If you're inspired to try and get to where I am, awesome, whether you have to use crutches to do it or you can barely walk anymore. I'm not breaking any speed records; in fact I think I might be getting slower, not faster. If you're inspired to stay faster than my molasses butt for your entire life, excellent. It's your inspiration and your path. No one can walk(run) it for you.

That trail ain't gonna run itself!

McCollum Park. Day eighteen. You'll recall McCollum is in Mill Creek, and I'm running from the park to Mill Creek Town Center again. Out and back this time, no pick up from my friend the police Officer today. Thebike path winds through the picturesque woods. The whole path is bordered by a native growth area.

My new pre-run routine(as of right now, because I just thought of it) is to try to clear my mind of all these expectations I haven't been able to shake. I don't know why I start out my run with all these expectations of accomplishment. So now I try not to do that. I'm just going to run. No PR, no record-setting anything. Just a run. That way I'll be able to detach myself from the outcome. This run should be a good one: I know the course, the distance, so I don't have to watch the clock for any reason. We ran this course two times a week a couple summers ago, back when I had another brief flirtation with physical fitness.

30 minutes, fine. That's it.

Don't panic, Tony. Why does trying not to be nervous make me nervous?

This might not be a great pre-run ritual after all.

It's like the old trick: "Don't think of a pink polka-dotted elephant." Well of course now you're thinking of it. You can't NOT think of it. It's there, and trying not to think about it makes it more real. You have to replace the thought with something else. The brain works involuntarily most of the time.

I've got my weight locked down, apparently, at 242 pounds. Here's a hint. When the doctor recommends "diet and exercise," the "and" in that sentence is really important. It's not "diet OR exercise." Or "maybe diet, maybe exercise." It's both if you want to lose weight. I think that's finally starting to sink in. It would be nice to have an outcome in terms of weight management, as something to look forward to. Unless I'm willing to do the unthinkable and change my diet, I have to let that one go. Eighteen days in here, I have lost nary a pound. That's okay. Baby steps.

My wife's running four miles, and I'm running three or three and a half. I guarantee you she's going to beat me. Ugh, see I can't clear my head of this expectant mindset. Polka dot elephant, polka dot elephant.

The oscillation our mind experiences is staggering. I never really realized that. Far from being at peace, my mind is always moving, always fighting itself.

I walk for ten minutes. My watch isn't linking up. I'm about ready to pitch this thing into the woods. It's messing with my mojo.

(Author's note: the author has no mojo. He's just blaming everything but himself now.)

I decide to use my stopwatch. I have all of my wife's hand-me-down watches in addition to this one(a birthday gift), so I resolve to strap on one of the other ones on next time as backup. I get all my wife's hand-me-downs, including my first iPod. Everything except the boots, of course. Wrong shoe size. That's a shame too because I can rock the pumps.

Not too sore today, another encouraging sign. My body is coping with this experiment in a way I had not anticipated. Our bodies really are made for running.

This run has one major hill feature about halfway in. I run to that hill – downhill going this direction - lost in my thoughts, almost like I forget what I'm doing. I really like that feeling. There's truly something magical in ignoring your watch.

I pass my wife on her return trip, and give her a "high-five" as we pass. I'm far behind her pace, of course. What's funny is that whenever we pass, I hold my hand out to give her a high-five. She always misses it. I have to ask her about that. It's like dumb and dumber out here with the high-fives. Guess which one I am?

Mid-point for me, the turnaround. I've run the whole time. I allow myself a little latitude in case I want to stop, but keep chugging along.

I'm enjoying a nice thought buffet today, and everything seems orderly about it. One fun thing to think about after another, my mind is rife with ideas.

## The One Religious Thing I'll Say

Not to get all religious on you, but I believe that nosehairs and those little hairs that grow on your *ears*, together, are a pretty convincing argument *against* the existence of God. I mean, I would like to talk to God and see what those things are for, purpose-wise. On the other hand, God works in strange and wondrous ways, so we probably shouldn't question this. He might be really sensitive about it, and he's done some pretty terrible things to unbelievers over the years.

The trail back is just a tiny bit uphill, so not much hope for a negative split. Still, I have that almost elated feeling. Quitting is optional. I'm very much in charge of moving my legs as far as I want to move them. A heron flies overhead, its feet tucked behind it, little heron toes splayed out. The heron in flight is actually pretty majestic, toes and all.

Let's see if I can make it up this blasted hill. My body(mind, really) is screaming for a walk break. I don't know the time and I won't look and you can't make me. I challenge myself to run up it.

There was a time when the idea of making it up this hill was laughable. But today, I crush it.

I pass an older gentleman walking up the hill, but just barely pass him. I make it up the hill by slowing wayyyy down. I wasn't running much faster than he was walking.

At the top I give myself a one-minute celebratory walk break. Who cares, so what. I still own this run.

My feet are feeling a little bit sore. I'll have to watch that and ice them tonight.

I take my second watch break at the place where I started my run, a fork in the trail, which is still probably a half-mile away from the car. I'll just do a walk/run back to the car and call it a day. A really strong, fun day.

Can I share with you the biggest surprise to me in this experiment? Yes Tony, please do – we're already reading your damned book, don't be holding out on us. The biggest, most surprising benefit I am experiencing is dictating my thoughts during a run and making sense of them on paper. It's a dialogue with myself where I witness my own highs and lows, my own flashes of brilliance and my idiotic dumbassery. I can take unrefined thoughts and refine or discard them, and re-live and re-experience my run each day. Its crazy refreshing. Crazy refreshing and also a bit crazy crazy.

It's an immense help to track and record my progress. I get the inescapable feeling that I am moving, growing. It's therapy. I find what moves me, what drives me, what stops me.

Yes, running is therapeutic. Like electroshock. Waterboarding might be more apt. Some combination of therapy and torture.

Recording my thoughts has been a wonderful experience. I would only caution that if you're dictating thoughts while running and you run up next to someone sitting in a chair behind a stump where you couldn't see them, and they have probably been listening to you talk to yourself for a few seconds, just GO WITH IT. Pretend you're on the phone with someone. Heck, they don't know. That was slightly embarrassing.

I'm back to the park now, and I see my wife making what is probably her 718th lap around the park's perimeter. She's cooking. I fall in line some twenty meters behind her. Can I catch her?

Uh, nope.

That's clear when I kick it into gear for another twenty yards and make up absolutely none of the distance between us. I tuck my tail between my legs and cut across the softball field towards the car. She still beats me. It's not close. I might as well have raced an airplane.

I finish the run with a thought about my own competitiveness. That competitiveness may be nothing more than insecurity. I try hard because I want to represent that I am better than I am, in relation to whatever metric I am concerning myself with. I am better than I was, I am better than that person, I am better than this time. All of these things are artificial measures, but paramount to a low self-image that has to succeed. I have always considered myself someone without too much of an ego, but running exposes me for an over-competitive fraud.

I am not saddened by this realization. I am strengthened by it.

## Day 18 Results:

Weight: 242
Miles: 3.26 (mapmyrun)
TOF: 35 minutes, 46 seconds
10:59 average pace
Mood: Strong.

## 19. "IF IT WASN'T FOR THE COFFEE, I'D HAVE NO IDENTIFIABLE PERSONALITY WHATSOEVER." – DAVID LETTERMAN

I make my wife mad.

If you are married to someone for a long time, you begin to develop the ability to push all of their buttons. It's not intentional. Sometimes it's just a reflection of where your relationship is at, or a boiling over of pet peeves. Living together can be difficult, especially when patience wears thin. And you know, we have three children. So patience can wear thin.

A month ago my wife asked me where her favorite coffee cup was. I didn't know. I suspected. But I didn't know.

Then came the searching, through every nook and cranny of the house. The garage. Outside. In the cars. Nothing.

I apologized: I feared I had lost it. I feared that I had taken it on one of my many summer trips to Home Depot and put it down while looking at a piece of lumber, or a type of lacquer, or variety of twine. I do think that's probably what happened. That mug is still at-large.

My wife was very upset at this mug's loss. She's had it for years, a hand-crafted mug that I think she bought at a craft show.

And guess what I did yesterday? I broke her second-favorite mug, an "I <3 NY" mug that we bought when we visited New York with the kids a few years ago, with a heart in the middle. I swung a bag of groceries over the cup and set it down on the handle. Snap.

I am the master of mug disaster.

I'm also in the doghouse for other reasons. As I said, I work in business marketing, but lately the pickings have been thin, so that tightens the budget, and led to some shall we say "points of discussion" in our house.

A cup isn't love, of course, and neither mug is(or ahem, *was*) as important as our relationship. But that's a false equivalency and I know it. Breaking them still makes her furious.

What is love?

(If you read that and the next words out of your mental mouth were "baby don't hurt me," then I consider you a friend.)

But as long as we're thinking of love, what do I expect to experience from running? Do I expect my relationship with running to be romance, wine, and poetry? Will I be writing poems to running? Do I expect a never-ending honeymoon with running? Or do I expect to have a tumultuous relationship, full of joys and sorrows – like my marriage?

In the news this week Charles Manson got engaged. If someone can fall in love with Charles Manson, can't I fall in love with running?

Of course, I began this challenge thinking of puppy love. An immature, fairy tale love, instead of what I know in my heart love is – something that matures, that definitely has its moments of grandeur, but also staggers sometimes.

A lot like me when I run.

Guess what I'm getting my wife for Christmas? Love. Lots of love. And probably a couple of personalized coffee mugs. I'm considering these:

"Someday this cup will break. Get over it."

"If this cup breaks, call 1-800-divorce for an attorney near you"

"Caution: contents may be hot. Holder of cup is hotter."

"No coffee is as strong as my love for you. (No coffee mug, either)"

Of course I'm leaning towards one of the last two. Because I may be an idiot, but I'm not that much of an idiot. If we meet someday and you remind me of those other mug sayings, I will disavow all knowledge of them. Especially if I am with my wife. And if you bring them up, we can no longer be friends, and your earlier recognition of "Night at the Roxbury" means nothing.

A little soreness in my back today, a twinge in my little toe, and a knee that feels slightly stiff. Issues I have been remarkably free from. If I end up losing a toenail or two, that would be marvelous.

"If my feet are sore running for three miles, then after a half-marathon they will be hamburger," I think lamely. Also I am hungry all of a sudden.

Running on a trail is my prescription for my slight soreness; I sagely advise myself to run on a trail rather than on a bike path, because I have no medical training at all and don't know what I'm talking about in any way.

I'm going to Willis Tucker Park today, east of Mukilteo in Snohomish County, south of the city of Snohomish, north of Bothell, east of the sun and west of the moon.

It's an 80 acre park with a mile-and-a-half trail around the perimeter. It's not a nature preserve, or a trail system, or an estuary. It's a park. It has a nice playground with a water feature for the kids. Baseball fields. That sort of park.

I'm fortunate so far in that I haven't run the same trail more than a couple times. That's going to change here as I wind up the experiment, of course, but it has been nice to get out and discover what is practically in my backyard.

Willis Tucker is about ten miles away from my house, and as I travel there I reflect on my hope for another good run. I've had a series of invigorating experiences running over the last few days, and I hope that continues. I'm pleased with that, and the fact that while I'm not gaining in speed, I am at least gaining... power, might be the best way to describe it. I seem to be "getting into it" more, enjoying it more. And here I go again using words like "enjoying" while talking about running. It's true; I'm finding a lot of strength in this exercise and gaining in power from it.

I have an op-ed piece coming out in our little hometown newspaper today, the Mukilteo Beacon.

Sometimes you fight in your life to find the things that you want to do, but the only way you know you want to do them is that you keep coming back to them. It's not so much a passion as it is a natural affinity. You default to them. You find meaning in everything else through them. For me, that's not running – at least not historically, though will that change? For me, it's writing. I'm not sure when that started. It might have started when I started writing book reports on notecards in my room in the fourth grade. Or when I wrote bad poetry for all those years after college. In college I cranked out three to five page reports over and over again. I probably five to ten papers per year, and I was good at it. I really thrived on it. In a way, it helped me organize, make sense of the world.

Writing in your job, for an actual living, though, that's a rarer thing. And I have a facility with people, so I went into sales for years. There was little writing, unless it was writing powerpoint presentations, or a newsletter, or a training manual for those that followed me. I tried to write a short story or two, but it seemed directionless to do so. I came to the conclusion that I'm not a writer.

So I ignored the thing I loved. Actually, I assumed that writing, and the love of writing, was a phase I went through.

If you stop doing the thing you love, then the world makes less sense.

In a very real way writing is my way of understanding things a dialogue with myself.

So it feels a little bit like a homecoming today, having a little slice of writing get any kind of validation. And that is part of my strength today, too. A return to what I know that writing this book represents. Running is a bit of an accident in this way – it could be exactly what I needed to spur me forward.

Running gives me the power I need to rediscover what I love.

I drive across the Boeing Freeway(Highway 526), and I see the panorama of the Cascade mountains ahead. Have I convinced you to move yet? This is stunning, the jagged peaks in the distance. It's hard to imagine that you could live around consistently beautiful scenery like this. I'm on a freeway and it's spectacular. Yay Pacific NW. Thanks for being your beautiful self.

Well now that I've regaled you with tales of love, it's time for a run. That will definitely take me down a couple notches. Even a good run is a challenge, so I don't want to get ahead of myself and assume everything will be amazing. Running is still absolutely a challenge, even on my best days.

That's the way life is, isn't it? A bit of success, a bit of recognition is all well and good, but you have to take the good with the bad. So I'm prepared to go out and suck some more today in an attempt to get to any piece of meaning.

Willis Tucker Park sits in a really nice neighborhood for running, with nice wide streets with large borders and sidewalks on both sides. It's really a runner's dream neighborhood. As I pull in I see another trail or two in the adjoining woods. All those sidewalks and they have trails through the woods also? Wow.

I start at the bathroom. I'm pretty sure that's what real runners do, start at the bathroom. In fact, I think the bathroom is part of the run.

I've got my two-watch backup plan going, which looks ridiculous. The old Forerunner watch finds the satellite immediately and the Nike+ Sportswatch cycles to find the satellite, but fails to find it. Surprise! Problem confirmed.

Here's an example of people not wanting to change their behavior. Remember when I mentioned how nasty coffee burps were? Well, rather than changing my own behavior and stopping my coffee consumption, I just change the way I drink coffee. Instead of a Chai Tea Latte, which gave way to nasty burps, I stopped earlier and got a Peppermint Mocha. Hopefully that will have nice energizing, refreshing burps. Isn't that just an elegant solution?

The hardest part of a run is the first five minutes. Going from inertia to running seems to shock the body. Sometimes I feel almost instantly fatigued. If you are going to run, you have to fight through that moment. Three minutes in, my body screams "STOP!" I keep punishing it.

I take a right out of Willis Tucker after a teensy weensy one-quarter mile loop, back on the main drag to hit that adjacent forest trail I noticed on the way in. It dives into the woods for a half a mile, and it's just fantastic.

Ha! This little makeshift trail goes down and down and down. I'm making a tough climb on the way back, but I appear to be winding around the back of Willis Tucker on a trail I never knew existed. I hope that this somehow wraps all the way around and I'm not on some wild goose chase.

What sounds to be a big dog yawps from behind a fence. I take my headphones out, just in case poochie can get out. I am reminded again why some people don't like running in the woods – but I think it's wonderful. Especially if you go to a place where there aren't any significant safety concerns, or you can run with a small pepper spray in your hand.

This is a really enjoyable trail, but it ends abruptly at a small unused park. I stop to do a few pull-ups.

Okay, one pull-up. News flash: running does not build your biceps. Owch.

I'm across a ravine and on the other side of Willis Tucker, so I keep moving in a direction that looks like it might someday take me back. I keep bearing right and end up climbing up to an apartment complex.

Note to self: million dollar idea! A hat that looks like a satellite dish, would also keep water off your head. Instant satellite linkup. Could also make it a Wifi hotspot!

I have no idea where I am, and I hope I don't have to loop back the way I came. I end up in an apartment complex, looking behind it to where the park might be. I look down one row, no access. Another. Nope. Finally I spot a set of stairs between two apartments, so I take them and can see Willis tucker behind the complex through a six-foot chain link fence. I can either jump it or try to slither under. Dangit.

The fence has what appears to be a bend in it, so I head over thinking I might be able to jump over it more easily. And lo and behold, I have somehow picked the one place where the fence opens up. This fence is hundreds of yards long, and I happen to take the stairs up right next to the one break in the fence. Eureka!

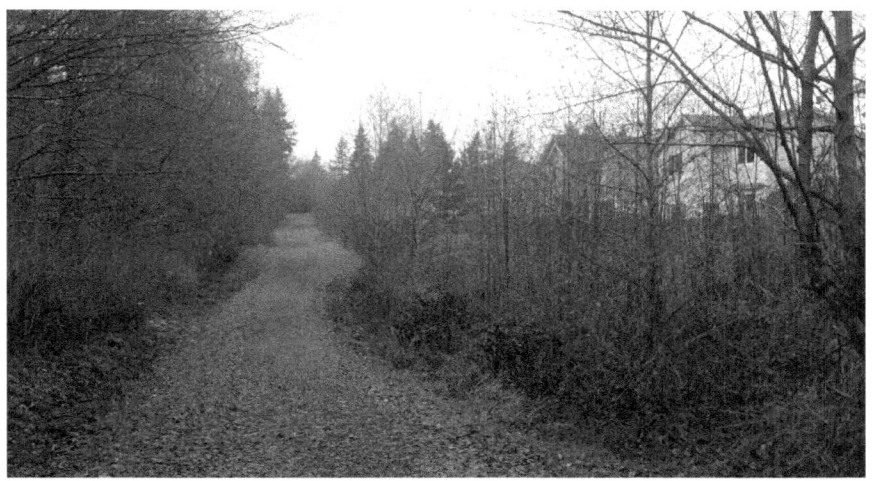

I'd rather be lucky than good, sometimes. I'm back in the park.

I loop around to the dog park, arguably the best feature of the park – though why anyone would want to argue about it, I don't know.

The dog park is probably six acres of fenced in area where dogs can roam and play. Even on a weekday like today there are around ten dogs with their owners playing, chasing balls, running with their tongues lolling out. A basset hound bays as he makes friends with a golden retriever chasing a ball. I can't help but chuckle. I run out to the street on the edge of the park and am greeted with the sounds of children playing at a school. Taking a right, I dip back to the park and run by owners with incredible dogs: a mammoth Rhodesian Ridgeback and two German Shepards, one with the more traditional whitish fur and black stripes and the other with that long, luxuriant black coat, combed to perfection. Their owners see me coming, look at the dogs, and laugh "who's walking who?" I smile back as I pass and say "They take you wherever they want to go." They laugh agreement.

I am back at the parking lot and I realize that my total time is over thirty minutes. My backup watch, the forerunner 305, has done well for me. The Nike never synched up. Stop paying attention to your watch and good things happen.

Today was a runner's run, if I do say so myself. I came out here and ignored the outcome. And if I can get myself to stop worrying so much about the outcome, that might be a victory in itself.

And by the way, the peppermint mocha burps were delightful, thank you for asking.

## Day 19 Results:
Weight: 244
Miles: 2.82 (mapmyrun)
TOF: 33 minutes, 43 seconds
11:59 average pace
Mood: This felt like I was a runner, just doing my running thang, burping peppermints, fa la la la la.

## The Runs

"I'm going running" and "I have the runs" are related sentences with completely different meanings.

It can't help our potential love for running that it's synonymous with diarrhea. In the spirit of fairness, let's apply similar counter-intuitive definitions to all sporting related activities.

"He's got a case of Soccer" shall henceforth mean the same as "he's overly dramatic and tries to get attention," a la the sport's main knock: pretending you were fouled. Example: *Glenn Beck has a bad case of Soccer.* Another acceptable use is a baby who bites someone to gain advantage. We can all thank Luis Suarez for that one.

Someone who is a "baseballer" has the tiring habit of overcomplicating things until they are so boring no one wants to listen. Like in baseball where there is one out, a man on second and the batter bunts to advance the runner, and the bunt goes right down the third baseline so the catcher has to run up the line, where he has a better angle at getting the leadoff runner, but has to make the decision on whether to pivot and try to get the hitter running to first even though he has a better angle at the leadoff man, which of course he would have to tag out. *YAWN* Get it? Also, the definition includes anyone who tries to describe the theories of Stephen Hawking. *Roy came to my party, but he baseballed until every other guest left.*

When someone says "I am going to try to Basketball this" he means he waits until the very end of regulation to put in his best effort. It shall be synonymous with procrastination and "sandbagging" until the end of the time allotted. *Cheryl partied all semester and then tried to basketball her way through finals week.*

If someone looks at someone and says "That guy plays football" then he is saying that person is a bully. Or that person is a felon. For instance: *Michael Vick plays football.*

Okay, not all of them are counter-intuitive.

## 20. "FREEDOM FROM MENTAL DISTRACTION EQUALS POWER" – DAN MILLMAN

The internet delighted me this morning. It wasn't anything as inane as lolcatz, those are so stupid. I hate those.

It was loldogs.

A Jezebel video proclaimed: "This golden retriever is learning a very valuable lesson way earlier than most of us do: sometimes you are just f#$@ng terrible at something and that's that."

The video, which looks like a Swedish-made doggy version of *America's Got Talent*, features dogs passing an "agility" test, which isn't really an agility test at all. It's a test of focus, if nothing else. Dogs are required to sit at the start, and then, when signaled "go" by their owners, have to run to them at the other end of a short runway. Sounds easy!

The catch is that there are treats. Delicious sausages, squeaky toys are on either side of them on the runway. Canned food. You have to admire the discipline as one by one, the dogs advance through this gauntlet of distraction.

Until the golden retriever. At whatever the Swedish word for "go" is, this furry guy gets about halfway down and wakes up. He wakes up to the possibility surrounding him. And though his owner calls urgently for him, damned if that isn't the best thing he's ever tasted right there. And this ball, you see, let's give that a squeeze. And apparently I missed some, I'm going back for this other dish. Is this a buffet? Sausage too?!

Benny Hill music plays. His owner looks angrily on, but our new favorite dog has a purpose. As determined as other dogs were to finish the course, he's determined to finish the food. All of it.

I admire that dog in one way: he got chow. Other dogs got nothing. Except inner peace.

I'm over halfway down this path, this experiment, and I've successfully ignored the distractions. I have to be honest and say I am pretty surprised at that, because in life I am totally golden retriever about this type of thing. Squirrel!

Big Gulch run today. Does it feel like a chore? A little. On day one, it felt like a chore, despite my excitement. It still feels like that, twenty days in. I guess I have to warm up to it.

I'm not feeling like "I will lace up for GLORY!"

It's more like "Well. Let's get this done." And that's a relatively positive outlook, probably owing to my ongoing expectation that I will actually do just that. Just under three miles. I'll set my watches and won't look. Cross my heart. It doesn't matter. If you're doing what I used to do and set time distances, where you can say "I should be here by 9:30, and this far by 22:00," that's not something that helped me EVER. Often as not, it became a source of frustration.

Again, running. No expectations except to run.

I figured out how to warm reboot my nike+ sportwatch, so I put it next to my Forerunner watch and try to link them both up. I zip up my rainproof vest, and *boom* the forerunner wins the linkup competition handily. The nike+ watch doesn't link. Sigh. Time for a factory reboot.

I snake my headphones up under my shirt – woo! That's cold. It's an overcast, cool day, not freezing. But the winds were whipping along this morning. The sky looked like a commercial, with the clouds flying past at fast forward.

I start my run at 1:00pm. Thank goodness there are downhills early on this run, because at 1:03 I am sucking air. Inertia. I'm discovering why my wife always starts slow.

At the four minute mark, I take a break at the hillside vista over Puget Sound. I can see the ferries in the distance, heading from Mukilteo to Clinton on Whidbey Island.

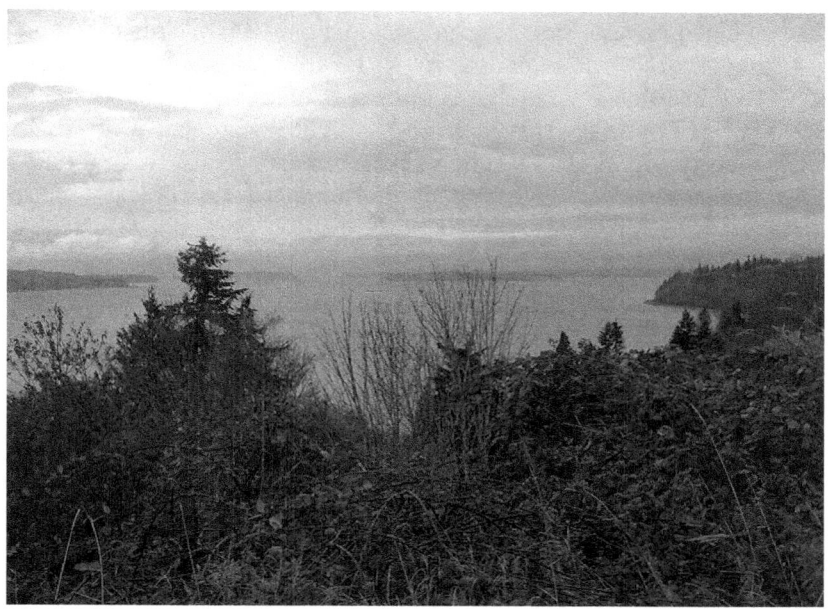

I hit my stop watch again after a picture break and press on. Does that count as stopping? Do I need to start over? Shut up. It counts. Don't be ridiculous.

I stop well in advance of my normal stop, not even to the bottom of the hill. There's a mid-point with a slight uphill, and I'm totally gassed, probably because I'm blazing along at breakneck speed – probably a twelve minute mile! Hold up there Usain Bolt. Leave something for the end there, speed demon.

For a guy with this much hot air, you'd think I wouldn't run out of breath so easily.

When I was a kid, I used to get these awful earaches when I ran; the wind would whistle in next to my eardrum and make my ears sore. Since I started wearing headphones, I don't have that problem. That and the fact that I am running half as fast. Actually, now that I think of it, the speed probably doesn't have anything to do with it. Totally unrelated.

Yeah, you read that correctly. I used to run so fast I would give myself an earache!

"What the heck happened old man?" *shakes fist barmily*

Bah. Kids today with their quicker paces. All over my lawn.

I run to the bottom of the hill at mile one and start towards the uphill section. I have my second walk break before the hills, so I start talking to myself immediately. I'm not looking at my watch, but I have to ask myself what the difference is? Why do I have so much less wind today than I've had in other runs? It's going to be one of *those* runs.

And yet, even if it's not as great so far from an aerobic perspective, I don't fear it. I don't dread the rest of the course even though I'm clearly not doing well so far. That might be a slight difference, which is likely related to my success so far. I don't feel trepidation, just frustration.

On the second set of switchbacks, another walk break. I can talk about walk breaks some more since I feel so compelled to take one. Obviously that makes me an expert on walk breaks.

It's like a fight in my mind as I run.

"You should stop now"

"Why should I?" (From my kickass, optimistic, Tony Robbins self)

"Because you're tired. You should stop"

I keep running, and Tony Robbins answers

"Yeah, but you're still running."

But that little voice doesn't go away. It just becomes more insistent, it crescendos, like that whining four-year old you try to have patience for, but he's relentless, he won't let up and you're trying to drive but he won't let go of his questions.

"So help me if I have to stop this car.....!"

So I stop, after the feud reaches a fever pitch, to make it stop, to silence that voice for a freaking minute, just to mute the din. I'm not even sure if I need to stop anymore, but jumpin' jehosaphat, that guy wouldn't shut up.

What is it that makes us want to stop, that starts that voice in our heads? And how are so many people able to shut it off?

I had a phone interview today for a management position. During my interview I talked a bit about setting expectations with people as being the key to getting performance from them – at least initially. If your mind reports to you directly – as it's supposed to - then could the key lie in setting proper expectations for how far you run? I think about that subject sometimes, the idea of running as far as you are able – with the understanding that your mind sets the distance. How far can you run? Why do you think that? Is it possible you can run further than that but your mind is stopping you?

Today, I'm wasted. There are limits to what a motivational speech can do, to be sure. Some runs aren't going to be great. Whoops, I'm at the sewage smell. Have to run. And hold my breath. When thinking positive doesn't work, running from sewage does. TIP.

I'm halfway through on this run and I'm just feeling flat. The positive vibe I had going even after struggling up the first hill is gone, replaced by the sounds of air escaping my lungs and a low-energy level. If I was wearing an energy-o-meter it would be stuck on "meh." Keep an eye at your local bookstore for *Re-Run 2: I wear a heart monitor this time.*

The irony is that this is my normal run, the good run, the run by my house, the one I can do any time. So far, it's one of the worst days yet.

I am all golden retriever today. Head's not in the game. Not focused on the goal. Mama said there'd be days like this.

At least I can focus on nature. I focus on what's around me and notice an enormous cedar stump at mile two. I've run by it every time, but never really noticed how beautiful it is, covered in vines.

Hey, at least I can get some tree hugging in if I can't run for crap.

(Author's note: I did not actually hug the tree.)

I notice suddenly that as I dictate into my Olympus recorder on my run, my voice has gotten deeper. Since I ran awkwardly by someone hidden from view on the trail the other day, I suddenly sound like Christian Bale as Batman, like I'm talking into my glove and giving Alfred instructions to send the Batcopter to pick me up.

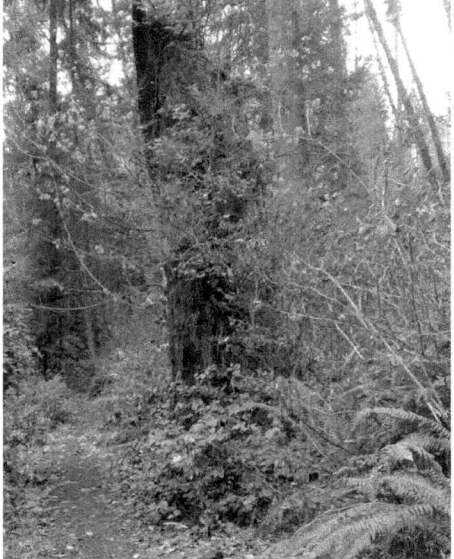

Wouldn't that be nice.

If it does take three weeks to make a habit, I'm on the cusp of making it a habit. This run makes me want to be on the cusp of giving up.

I've made a lovely walk break of this run. I come to the stairs fairly rested, so at least I can try to huff up those things.

I bumble up the stairs, making it halfway up.

At the top of the stairs is a wise old man(he has Beats headphones, so like, instant credibility). This is not fiction, it actually happened. He waits for me. I say "I'm not going to make it all the way up today."

He says "I try to make it here three or four times per week and do three iterations of those stairs. I was trying to make it to five, but I don't think I'll get there."

Good on ya, old feller. Keep fighting the good fight.

Did I just meet future me? I hope so. I seemed kinda kickass.

I come into 92nd Street Park through its nice log-framed entryway. I feel a tightness in my leg and my knee was a little wobbly up those stairs.

"The woods are lovely, dark and deep, but I have promises to keep, and miles to go before I sleep."

How awesome that poem, and yes, I am totally misusing it here. I have probably a half mile and then I can sleep, whenever. Yet today, it seems like I have so far to go before I'm finished. With this run. With this experiment.

I turn down the path to connect to the street. I mumble something into my recorder cursing my watch again, but I see something scurrying along the trail. Is that a rat? A mole? marmot? He staggers across the path. It's a fifteen-inch long critter with sleek fur, a blunt nose, and only a short tail. He seems to sense me for a moment, but he's too caught up in his own problems to concern himself with me. He gnaws on some leaves, stumbles this way and that. I take a few pictures, but he is in obvious distress.

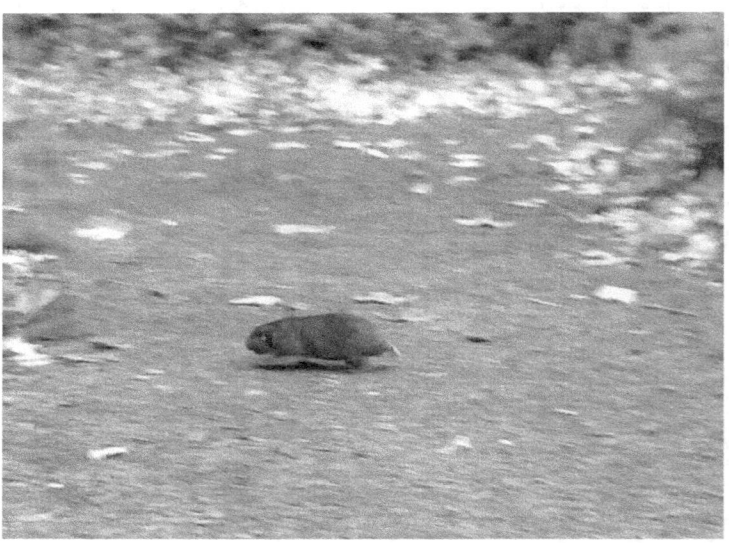

What do I do?

Well, I'm not going to pick the danged thing up. For all I know it's a mole someone poisoned in their yard. That seems rather likely, but he's just stumbling through the woods like a lost little red riding hood. It's quite sad, actually, and I can't make sense of it. He could recover, or he could be dead tonight. Did he eat the wrong mushroom? For all I know, he's gored and I can't see it. I leave him as he staggers off the trail and into the woods. He continues his journey. I continue mine.

I run/walk the last half mile troubled by thoughts of how my life isn't quite so bad, and wishing there was something I could do – thinking perhaps there was? I am unsettled.

It's surprising how a random thing like this affects you. Totally random. Can't make much sense of that, although I want to. I want to apply some knowledge, some meaning, recognize some pattern, but like the Golden Retriever all I see are things around me without any greater purpose than the moment. The Golden Retreiver got happy things, but I have a sad one, to go along with a sad run.

## Day 20 Results:
Weight: 241
Miles: 2.91 (mapmyrun)
TOF: 42 minutes, 00 seconds
14:25 average pace
522 Kcal
Mood: Hey, you know who has two thumbs and sucks at running?

## 21. "WE ARE WHAT WE PRETEND TO BE, SO WE MUST BE CAREFUL ABOUT WHAT WE PRETEND TO BE" – KURT VONNEGUT

*ChiRunning*, written by ultra-marathoner Danny Dreyer, is one of those books on getting back to the basics of running. As usual, I'm skeptical of some of the author's premises, but his results are undeniable. He's run 34 ultramarathons and has placed in fourteen of them. It's an inspiring story of one man's discovery of the principles of Tai Chi and how he applies them to run faster than I'd ever be able to run in my life.

Yeah, I'm starting it with the same reaction you probably just had: a lot of eye-rolling.

He notes the same thing I've experienced: that growing older means that suddenly we start to suck at running. Somewhere in our expedition through life, we forget what running is, and how to have fun at it. Our mechanics are completely screwed up by our life of bending over computer screens and walking in high-heeled shoes.

Hey, I can't wear flats to every society function, you know.

It's not that I don't recommend the book. Not at all. It's terrific. It's just that if I hear one more running coach talk about how they won so many races, I'm going to barf. Not because I don't respect that accomplishment, but it has little value for me, slug-slow runner than I am. I am more of an "Everyman" runner, so running fast at ridiculous distances doesn't really impress me in the same way that talking to the world champion of DanceDanceRevolution is inspiring, but also seems little crazy. And it doesn't excite me enough to go pick up the video game and try to compete.

Less soreness –and I'm on Day 21! I have to be proud of that.

My wife is off work today(a Friday), so we're going to Seattle for a run in Discovery Park.

She laughs at me as I get out of the car and start hooking up all my devices. My iPod clips on my belt-pack, my headphones to my ears. My recorder attached to my hand on a lanyard. Two watches. My phone goes in the belt-pack too. You can't make me call it a fanny pack. You can't make me! It's all slightly comical.

The Forerunner 305 wins the linkup contest. Again, it wasn't close.

I'm determined to hang loose today and just have fun. Yesterday sucked. I think we've established that. No further proof of suckage is required to make that case. Today I'm just going to let it flow and see where it takes me. Kind of a "When life hands you lemons" attitude.

I hate that saying. Make lemonade? What a trite, reductive saying. What if life gives you cancer? You can't make lemonade out of cancer. Horrible saying.

Or, in the words of Cave Johnson, a character in the videogame Portal 2:

"When life gives you lemons, don't make lemonade. Make life take the lemons back. GET MAD! I DON'T WANT YOUR DAMN LEMONS! WHAT AM I SUPPOSED TO DO WITH THESE?! DEMAND TO SEE LIFE'S MANAGER!"

A saying only a bit better: "Every cloud has a silver lining." I don't know who came up with that one, but it doesn't even make sense. Who has seen a cloud with a silver lining? What, are clouds suddenly made of fabric? Are clouds really pillows with a lining?

You might as well say "Every moon is made of green cheese."

Anyway, I'm going to make some, eh, er, lemonade or something. Make the run today better than yesterday. I don't know how. I'm just hopeful.

I tell my wife "I hope you don't mind running slow." And we take off.

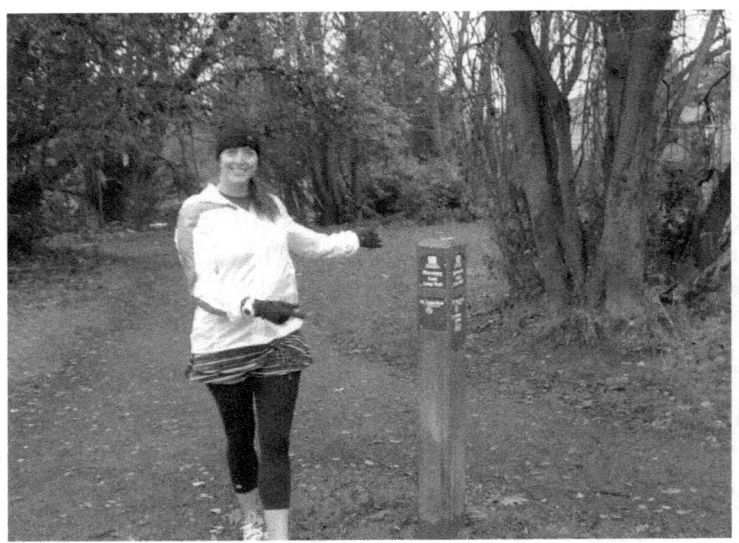

Ten seconds in, we're already lost. We're supposed to be on the 2.8 mile "loop trail," but it's pretty loopy and we lost it already. Oh well, we just continue on the perimeter of the park.

"Which way?" we ask a lot. My wife has run this before, but it's not like she's memorized the trail. We just generally track counterclockwise around the park's perimeter, hoping to catch the trail again.

I've lived in Seattle for more than twenty years, and it's only in the last couple of years that I've begun to explore the amazing outdoors we live in. Discovery Park is an amazing park in the Magnolia area of Seattle. Huge, old trees covered with lichen are all around this 534 acre park. We find the trail again and a simplified version of a map at another parking area.

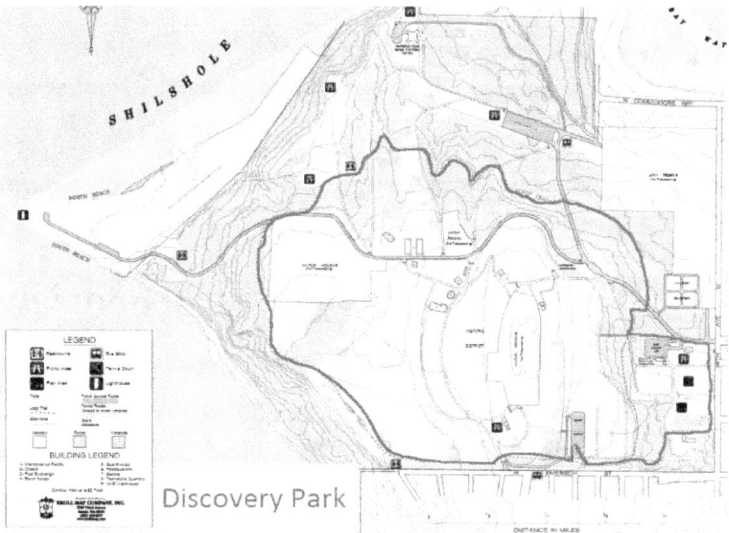

Discovery Park

It's a big park. You almost need to run with a guide.

We run a tunnel that I promptly dub "homeless tunnel" and the trail opens into more forest. I enjoy the view of a very typical PNW forest. Large, rangy oak trees among the pines, a huge amount of deadfall branches as ground cover. The branches provide a canopy up to thirty feet away from the trunk of the tree. Some very old trees here.

Fort Lawton resides in the middle of Discovery Park, a Fort that started in 1890 but it run by the city now. We don't run over there; I'm not sure any of the actual fort exists. We do see a well-maintained officers' quarters in the distance. As a strange side-note, my military training was at Fort Sill, Oklahoma, right outside the city of Lawton. Seems like an odd thing that I am destined to run around places named "Lawton."

I do enjoy the distraction of a trail run. Our trail is alternatingly mud, gravel, concrete sidewalk, and hard-packed sand as we come out on a bluff overlooking the sound. The distraction of running on a trail seems to help me to be more present in the run, enjoying it more, making the time go quickly.

My wife wants me to stay closer this run, just in case any weirdos are about.

I am passed by my wife when I take my second walk break at twenty minutes. I am saved by an off-leash dog, which causes her to pause and wait for me. He's friendly.

I started out well, but I'm running out of gas now. Come on!

I run by an older gentleman as I try to catch up to my wife. I say "she's winning, right?"

"Indeed," he replies.

I love that I live in a place where people say "indeed." It all seems so grown up around here.

It's raining in earnest now. I have that feeling of badassery that comes when the weather worsens, doing things no one else is dumb enough to do.

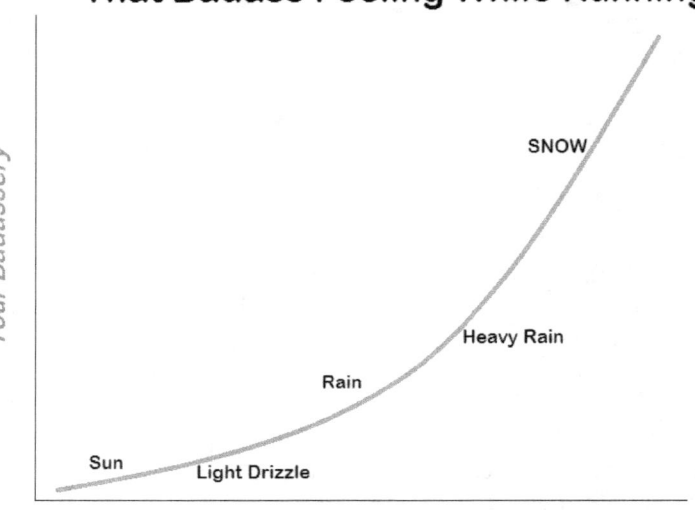

## That Badass Feeling While Running

*Your Badassery*

SNOW

Heavy Rain

Rain

Sun   Light Drizzle

*Amount of Precipitation*

Re-Run: My 30-Day Experiment to Fall Back in Love with Running

My wife is ahead of me now, but she loops back because there are a couple of unsavory middle-age characters ahead with poofy REI jackets and umbrellas, strolling along. I realize that most middle aged men with REI jackets aren't hardened criminals, but you never know. They might have also purchased a knife at REI, you see, and might be eager to recoup their investment on unwary passers-by.

She comes back for my accompaniment and a show of strength against the poofy jacket guys. Still, her having to circle back feels like she's babysitting me on this run.

The Puget Sound opens up before us as we run along a wide trail of gravel. Container ships move along shipping waterways.

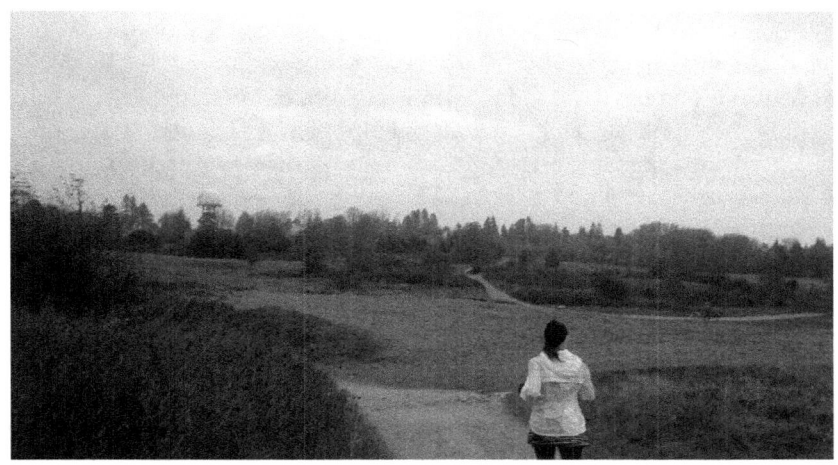

We plan to stop by the Brooks Running Outlet after the run today. The soles of my shoes don't look like they are totally broken down, but they might be the culprit behind my progressively sore feet, and they are feeling sore right now. Either that, or my mechanics are messed up, which is probably also true. Or I am doing something crazy and putting too many miles on my feet. That's also true. Still, I have had these shoes since July, and put a lot of miles on them with my 242 pound frame, so a shoe breakdown is imminent if it hasn't happened already. I would hate to be on the trail and have one of my shoes' have a blow-out. In an attempt to control my body, I would careen off a rockery and fall into a ditch, all because I didn't rotate my shoes adequately. Safety first.

I think about yesterday's run and the critter I saw. If you are familiar with the movie The Princess Bride, then you may recall the scene where a giant rat staggers into the Fire Swamp. I thought of that scene today as I recalled the random events of yesterday, with the marmot, or Nutria(River Rat), or whatever it was. It's like my memory creates a caricature of what happened, even a day ago. I suppose that seeing a large rodent in the woods might lead one right to that scene eventually, but I am still struck today with the idea that people try to make everything fit into some picture we have of the world. Everything must make sense. It's a cognitive distortion. Like trying to find meaning in running?

It's a way of making lemonade, and I seem to be making lemonade today, running and stopping but having a pretty solid run on the trail. A lot to see in Discovery park. I run past a large stand of light, airy pine trees at the top of the hill. These pine trees are more solitary in western Washington, but I've seen them all over the place as you cross the

Cascades into Eastern Washington. There are even a few of my favorite Madrona trees here.

It wasn't an easy run today by any stretch, but it went pretty quickly – so much to look at. That obviously helps. I felt fatigued in the middle, but it was manageable. A little foot pain. A nice run with my wife, and we head off to get a new pair of shoes.

## Day 21 Results:
Weight: 242
Miles: 2.99 (mapmyrun)
TOF: 35 minutes, 45 seconds
11.39 average pace
Mood: Give me enough nature to look at and I can run for longer!

I am weighing myself often to see if my weight fluctuates. It does, from 239 at the low to around 246 with clothes on. There's a pretty good range there, but my weight is not decreasing at all. When people train for a marathon, they don't lose weight: you work out more, you get hungry more, you eat more... and sometimes, you don't lose any weight. Your body balances it out. In fact, some people gain weight training for a marathon. I think we all hope our metabolism ramps up and we burn more energy. Doesn't always work out that way.

At the Brooks Outlet store I get a flashy new pair of yellow Glycerins, a tiny bit cheaper than the $110 we paid last time. I am totally stoked.

Speaking of ChiRunning, for lunch we go to "What the Pho" in Bothell. For lunch I order Pho "Tai Chin" and a sandwich with Taro fries. Which if you think about it sounds a lot like I ordered homeopathy with a side of superstition.

It is delicious.

# I do like my colorful pie graphs.

And here is a bar chart about my favorite pies:

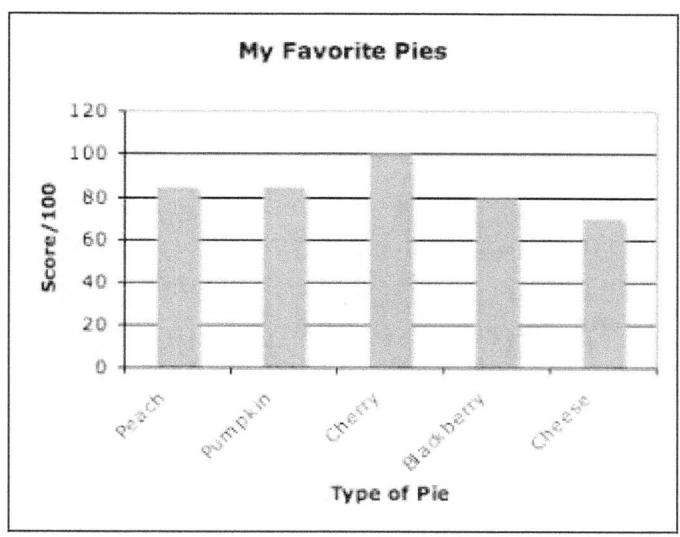

…and here is a pie graph of my favorite bars…

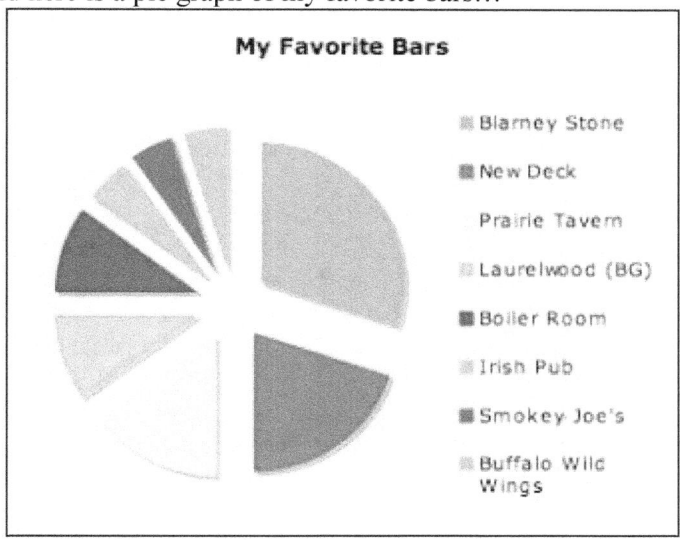

Some supreme geekdom there.

## 22. "SUCCESS IS THE ABILITY TO GO FROM ONE FAILURE TO ANOTHER WITH NO LOSS OF ENTHUSIASM" – WINSTON CHURCHILL

I'm going to keep failing…! At least for another eight days. My enthusiasm hasn't faded, though the bit of foot soreness lingers from yesterday, and it's rather hard to take that and feel excited about my run today.

Today I run with my middle son, who is twelve now and handsome as heck. Of my offspring, Aidan is more of a runner than the other two. The other two are athletic, to be sure, but Aidan has runner's legs and a natural flow and rhythm to his gait. Running also seems to suit his temperament. He hasn't played many team sports, so running Cross-Country seems to feed both his desire to be around other kids, still be on a team, but perform independently.

I mapped out a course from an intersection to our house, about three miles. We started this morning off watching our youngest son play soccer. They lost, spectacularly, but there were no tears, thankfully. On the way home, Aidan and I get dropped off at a gas station so we can start our run. It's pretty much a straight shot down the street on sidewalks all the way home for us.

Today is only slightly overcast, so both of my watches want to participate. I'm so glad you both showed up today. Harrumph.

I am faced with a conundrum. There is a Starbucks on the way, and it's against my religion to pass a Starbucks while running. It's sacrilege.

As I tell this to Aidan, I am suddenly comforted by the fact that I don't have my wallet. I will avoid cardinal sin today because Starbucks does not take payment in handsomeness. Neither my own nor my child's stunning looks will afford us a coffee, so until the opulence of Starbucks is converted to an appreciation for two sweaty yet undeniably handsome joggers, we run sans café.

I'm still a bit chilly from standing and watching a soccer game, but it's only 50 degrees or so out, and a tiny bit of sunshine leaks from the sky onto us. As we start, we warm up quickly despite our light shirts and shorts. Our hats help.

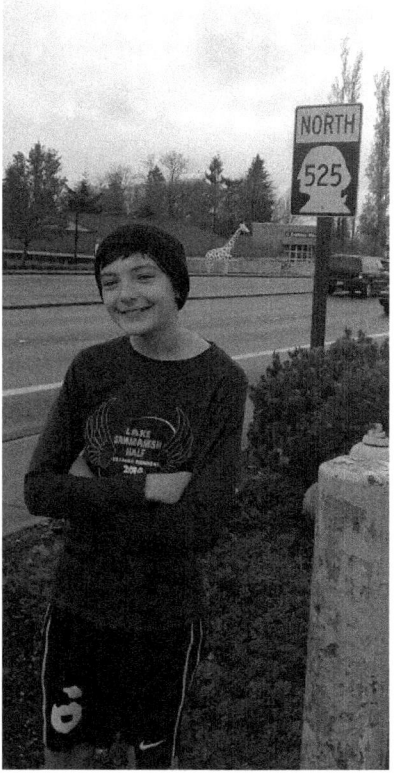

I have my new shoes on! Hopefully I can motor along in these things while my son bounds along beside me. Most of this run is slightly downhill.

I can't help but give my son running pointers. Like I'm some kind of danged expert. He has a bit of a torsional twist to his leg kick. If nothing else, it's definitely wasted motion. I'm a Dad. That makes me an expert in everything, doesn't it?

The only slowdown are the intersections where we have to wait for lights to change. Aidan sets a pretty killer pace for me. I hope I'm not being literal. I dare to glance at my watch, and it hovers around 9:00 for the first mile. This should be a pretty good run because I'm running with Speedy Gonzales. I suppose that makes me El Gato.

Instead of beautiful trees in the forest, as has been my norm, I run by a garage door service company. A Pet hospital. Lawn Equipment supply. Marijuana Dispensary. It's Washington.

My wife doesn't like running along this road; she feels like she is breathing in exhaust. I get it. There's no comparison to running through the woods and smelling fresh clean air. You can definitely tell when a diesel goes by. I am fortunate in that no one goes by me "Rolling coal," an exciting trend in our beloved southern states where you modify your diesel truck to spew MORE black smoke and then terrorize people by doing it next to them. Usually Prius owners, because everyone knows that Prius owners probably went to college and got all educayted and so they are the enemy. Also, they do it to runners.

Some people aren't content being stupid. They have to let everyone else know they are stupid. Rolling coal: a clear sign the apocalypse is upon us.

## "Keats and Yeats are on your side but you lose..." - The Smiths

I've been uncertain in most of this experiment. Uncertain if I should run with a goal, or without one, uncertain if I could like running, uncertain about why I don't like it. Uncertain if I should let go or hold on. Should I stay or should I go?

The poet John Keats described a principle he called "Negative Capability." I assume that I am capturing some aspect of this in trying to remain objective in my attitudes towards running. Keats described it this way:

"I mean negative capability, that is when man is capable of being in uncertainties, mysteries, doubts, without any irritable reaching after fact and reason."

In re-reading that, it is clear to me that is exactly the opposite of what I am doing. I am irritably "reaching after fact and reason", conclusion, meaning every day I am out here. I am struggling to make meaning of the world of running. That state of Negative Capability probably involves a whole lot more "being at peace" than I have been able to muster. Keats also said:

"...with a great poet the sense of Beauty overcomes every other consideration, or rather obliterates all consideration."

Obliterates all consideration? What the HECK John, I thought we were friends, and you betray me with this stuff about my sense of beauty. Or he could just be indicating that I am not a great poet.

I can live with that.

I am absolutely reaching after conclusion for this 30-day period. I'm searching for meaning, I'm hunting down the ambiguity of running so I can nail it to the wall. Keats indicated that was more Samuel Taylor Coleridge's style. So, I guess you could say I am more of a Coleridge than a Keats?

I can live with that too. In fact that's even better.

I actually like uncertainty. I like taking a problem and turning it over in my mind, examining it from all angles, even nonsensical ones. It's one of my key skills. It's often confused with indecision, but I like to weigh both sides of an argument. I'm one of the few people I know that is able to delay judgment. I think that's a holdover from my years in debate in high school. You had to be able to take both sides of an argument at will.

Pro and con. See them both. Solve for one. That carries over to today, where I often play the devil's advocate in a conversation, not to frustrate, but to explore something more fully.

That doesn't make me right, of course, any more than being a scientist makes you right on climate change. But with enough research and collaboration, and a preponderance of evidence and peer-reviewed literature, then we can indeed draw some conclusions. You eliminate bad data by having more data. In my case, that's a 30-day experiment. A week of running isn't enough to make a judgment, but 30-days and we have enough data points to start drawing generalizations, don't we? This is my own behavioral experiment.

And no, I'm not denying climate change. I'm saying that you need to research it to understand, but being in a position where you could research it doesn't make you right. Anti-vaxxers famously quote a study from Johns Hopkins stating that vaccines are of dubious value. Problem: The author, a Doctor, is a Doctor of anthropology. He's never done research at Johns Hopkins. His conclusions aren't peer reviewed; they are just observations.

Back to finding meaning for running: We need to snopes our life, you know? Draw conclusions based on a whole series of facts, not draw a line between a couple of data points and call it irrefutable proof of something. In my case, I loved running, then suddenly hated it. Did running change? Or did I change? And why would that decision be irrevocable? Just because I made a judgment doesn't make it true.

Except for the walk breaks waiting for the lights, we're keeping up a good pace this run. With a slight downhill for the rest of the run, this should continue to be a good one. Yeah, I'm looking at my watch, so what.

I talked a bit about running angry, and it worked. But the thing about anger is that it's not sustainable. It's not sustainable in a long run, and it's not sustainable in your life. There comes a time when you have to make peace with things, or you turn bitter, which turns to hatred. And then you end up being a 46 year old guy who walks around telling everyone "I hate running!"

The only way you can fall in love with something is to first make peace with it.

New shoes, yay, my yellow, grey and gold Glycerins. But boo: my feet are sore and uncomfortable. Break-in period? Sad face.

It's that nagging foot soreness, the feeling of compression on my arch that makes me want to take my first walk break. Aidan has been really good about bounding ahead and waiting for me, taking off, waiting. It's like me running with my wife.

"Aidan, do you remember a few years ago on my birthday you gave me a coupon for a free foot massage?"

"Yeah."

"I think I need to cash that thing in."

He smiles.

Ah, kids. As we pass the top of Hell Hill, at Big Gulch, I tell Aidan "if you really want to be strong, you should run down Hell Hill and back up the stairs near the park."

"Okay!" He nods enthusiastically, and he's off.

I'm left stammering as he leaps away down the path - "uh-uh-m-meet you at the playset!"

Kids and their play. It's just joy. It's just not work, to him. I'm here with sore feet, shuffling along, "gutting out" a run, and he's just enthusiastic about moving his body through space. He's not making some creepy decision to hate running.

I am definitely doing something wrong here. That little turkey.

I run into the park, past the top of the steps and wonder how far behind me Aidan is. He'd better not be in front of me.

I hear a loud clanging noise coming from the Gulch and double back to the steps.

Have you ever been running near your house, and an ambulance passes by, or a fire engine, and you have a moment where you think "Is that going to my house?" I have the same kind of feeling as my twelve-year-old runs through a park without me and I hear noises. He comes trotting out of the trail to the stairs, less than a minute behind me.

I am a little sad that my feet are sore. It's worrisome for more than today. This could sideline me, or at the very least make me miserable for the next eight days.

Aidan takes the lead through the park, running down the bark-strewn path and over roots. He has endless energy. He can't help but leap along like a gazelle. It reminds me of a show our family adores, "American Ninja Warrior," a show where contestants take on a series of physical obstacles trying to get to the final test, an obstacle course called "Mount Midoriyama." We love the show, and I am reminded of it as Aidan springs through the forest, reminiscent of some of the videos of contestants who are Parkour enthusiasts.

Aidan comes out on the sidewalk, still in the lead, and says "Finish Strong!" He takes off.

AAAAH! I hate it when they throw my motivational quotes at me.

We finish strong together.

Later, I realize that in my fit of cleaning my desk off I threw away my coupon for a free foot massage. I take a bath to soak away my troubles as best as I can. Is there anything that makes you a runner more than having a "nagging" injury?

## Day 22 Results:
Weight: 243
Miles: 3.1 (mapmyrun)
TOF: 34 minutes, 58 seconds
11:15 average pace
Mood: A tough but manly run with my son.

## 23. "THE FIRST TIME I SEE A JOGGER SMILING, I WILL CONSIDER IT." – JOAN RIVERS

Last night my wife and I went to a lovely dinner at a restaurant in Bothell.

We sat next to the guitar player Mike Bucy, who was very enjoyable. RIGHT next to, as in I flipped the pages for him as he played "American Pie." He played a mix of songs that favored James Taylor in a big way.

I expressed my frustrations to my wife about trying to find happiness in running – like Aidan had demonstrated, so naturally. I'm so attached to what I'm doing, to succeeding in it, that I can't enjoy it. I'm like a guy who dates women with the sole purpose of getting laid: so concerned with the outcome he can't enjoy the process of meeting people. Or falling in love.

My wife shared that running has "deconstructed" her – it's broken her down and allowed her to build herself up. She's worked out presentations, had epiphanies about what to work on at work, confronted herself, and found peace from everything that has frustrated her.

Well that all sounded lovely. It really sounded lovely after a couple of glasses of Pinot Gris.

I wake up today feeling more aches and pains. Not just from the wine, but that certainly doesn't help. I feel crapulous. Tightness in my calves, that crinkly out-of-sync feeling in my back. Foot soreness remains. Even my ankles feel crusty; I have to move them to break off what feels like a shell of plastic that encases them. Is this is the wall I was fearing?

The book ChiRunning contributes to this sinking feeling. The author talks about developing that youthful joy while running as an adult. There's bad news here too: the process of doing that can take years. Of course that's true. It is naïve of me to think it would be simple, unrealistic to expect that I would go out for a run for a few days or a few dozen days and suddenly find myself joyful, isn't it?

I don't want to take years. Runners are supposed to be patient. Well, I'm not. I want to enjoy it and I want to enjoy it now. I demand that I enjoy it. I grasp after happiness and come up empty, time and again. I strive to understand, but it's a process that only leads to more questions.

I am miserable and being dropped off on the side of the road.

It's another sidewalk run today, like yesterday, a sidewalk drop by my wife. I have no idea if I'm going to fall on my face today. I'm tired enough that I start my run by not running. By walking. Taking it slow, just getting my mileage in.

This is the first day I have dreaded the run. It isn't just that obligatory 'I have to do this' feeling. I really don't want to.

I feared some kind of wall. This must be it. Obviously my mechanics need some help, because I'm experiencing some breaking down physically. But I'm out here today to finish the job. If the spirit of running is to die within me, then I want to be merciful and end put it out of its misery quickly. If it is meant to rise from the ashes like a phoenix, then I want to get to that point as soon as possible.

So I start at a nice 11:00 pace, nice and easy so I can keep it going.

I plotted this run on the map as a drop-off, like yesterday. My son is playing in a soccer tournament, so I have my wife drop me off here, about three miles away so I can run to the game. It's on arterial roads with good sidewalks. Flat level run. And I have a break in the clouds and a sunny day. Thank goodness for that. If today was the day I get freezing rain? I shudder.

The sun feels good.

Today is warm enough, in fact, that I don't need any kind of outer layer. I bring a hat because it's mid-afternoon and the temperature will start cooling off in awhile. Other than that I am lucky to be able to wear shorts and a thin long-sleeved technical shirt.

It's been a long time since I felt any spinal problems, but today I feel that tightness in the mid-upper back, caused by what? Running mechanics or sitting hunched over a computer screen. That tension arrests me initially and I try to relax through it. For the first mile it's a jogalittlewalkalitlejogalittlewalkalittle kind of run. Craptastic.

I jog by a Target shopping cart parked by the sidewalk. We're almost three miles from the nearest Target. Shopping cart = homeless RV.

## Charles Darwin: not a runner

Through this experiment, it occurs to me, I might be denying my future offspring a strong foothold in evolutionary development. If I keep running, working out, I am feeding the human ability to run, then it's possible that my children, my children's children, and my children's children might develop an even greater capacity for running. They might evolve greater ability. Of course in modern society the ability to think and work through problems is most valued. So by working against that idea, I may be cheating future generations of more intellectual-based gifts. I may be holding civilization back! I may be contributing to the fall of society by running *today*.

Listen, if you want a real reason to not run, there ya go. Try this at a cocktail party when someone asks if you run:

Them: "Do you run?"

You: "Of course not?"

Them: "Why not?"

You: "My life is dedicated to helping my progeny advance evolution in the areas that hold the greatest human potential. Science. Philosophy. The Arts. I would no rather encourage a child or myself to run than I would teach them to attack an animal with spear made of bone."

Something like that. And be sure you say all that LOUDLY and with disdain in your voice. Let me know your results! Please email me. PLEASE, I mean it.

Here's a "silver lining" on a difficult day. On a day like today I have an incredible capability to defend the premise that running is stupid.

At the mile and a half point, I figure the only thing that can save me is doing fartleks. So I proceed to run to a pole, and then take a walk break. Pick out a pole in the distance somewhere, run to it and take a walk break. As I try to run this way, I try to open up the throttle on my speed, which is a bit *more* painful. Even for that small interval, the pain in my legs and feet increases as I try to improve my kick, both to the front and to the rear.

My kick is kicking my ass.

My top speed is a 7:40 mile though. That is, my top speed doing fartleks for probably a hundred yards.

It's in these moments of pain that I realize that I need to revisit the diet conversation. Carrying around 244(today) pounds of weight is challenging. Carrying 220 would be at least 90 percent of the effort, ten percent easier. I could use that ten percent right now. I resolve to try to watch it a little more from here on out. Eight days remain – with a half-marathon – but I can take it easy and not eat my normal six slices of cheesecake every day, right?

Author's note: I don't think that is humanly possible to eat six slices of cheesecake. I like cheesecake but I don't think I've even had a slice of cheesecake in a few years. I think my point is that I will try to be more moderate in my eating habits.

My wife and I had a beautifully prepared dinner last night. I had a Filet Mignon, well done but still tender, mashed potatoes and green beans. A lovely pinot gris. It was fantastic. But if you're trying to lose weight, you need to spend a tiny bit more time on those considerations. A little less chips. I little less beer. A little more carrots would do wonders, not only for my physique, but also for my ability to run.

Around mile two the pain subsides a little bit. At least, I'm able to block it out. That may be my only hope in the half-marathon – running through the pain. At this point I am able to kick it into gear for –oh gosh - it must be almost a half mile without much pain. I'm spectacular.

I dare a glance down at my watch, confirming my pathetic pace, and also confirming that I'm almost done. Wow, that sucked, but I didn't fall flat on my face. In fact, I didn't even stumble.

Running and snow and rain might make you feel badass, but the ultimate is running in pain. For those of you runners who run in pain, you are way baddasser.

Yesterday, running with Aidan was like two boys running. Aidan at twelve and me at an age no one could remotely consider boyish unless you use that to describe the experience in a strained analogy. Today is all responsibility, all grown-up work and hatred. Honestly, I expected to be here ten days ago. Now the challenge is on, and we'll see what the next eight days bring. I remind myself that the phoenix had to be lit on fire before it was able to arise from the ash. Today marks one or the other: the start of a transformation or the first day of being lit on fire.

## Day 23 Results: "Way to get out there"
Weight: 244
Miles: 2.95 (mapmyrun)
TOF: 35 minutes, 26 seconds
12:38 average pace
522 kcal
Mood: If Frank Frazetta drew runners, there would be a picture of me somewhere fighting off a giant snake with an axe, covered in scratches. A few bite marks. Some blood. In metaphor, that was this run.

## 24. "SURPRISE IS THE GREATEST GIFT THAT LIFE CAN GRANT US" – BORIS PASTERNAK

The day comes like the first day I started this experiment, full of promises and broken dreams, heavy with anticipation and a touch of dread. I have six days left, my feet aren't bloody, but I'm sore enough to question my sanity. Again.

I am gathering my energy to fight valiantly this day, to take up the sword of fitness and slay the demons of sloth. I am focusing my energy on getting through my run and experiencing the highest of holy pilgrimages this day.

The journey to the blessed hot tub.

I finally had a brilliant idea that I would soak away my troubles and try to experience nirvana by going to the YMCA. Can't hurt.

Okay, I lied. It wasn't my idea. It was my wife's idea. Again, if you're just tuning in – she's the smart one.

It is a bit of an odd Monday. I had a two-hour chat with three different representatives from Comcast, solving almost nothing. I had a phone interview that got rescheduled until next week. It's mid-afternoon by the time my wife and I head out to the place with a song named after it. The eponymous YMCA. My wife will do some strength training, and I will run around the neighborhood and collapse in the hot tub. That's the plan.

Question: If you exercise to work out your problems and confront your demons, can you just call it "Exorcising"?

It's a more-than-typical Seattle day with a blanket of grey in the sky. The rain is typically Seattle too, the incessant drip drip drip that keeps the street wet but is barely worth an umbrella. Today it's a little more rain than that, so an umbrella is worth it. While we're on the topic, I hope those goofy little umbrella hats make a comeback, because those things were dorky, but still very handy. Some things are too stupid looking to take seriously, and I've always thought the little head umbrella deserved another shot at fame. Suggestion: not so rainbow-y this time. That could not have helped early adoption.

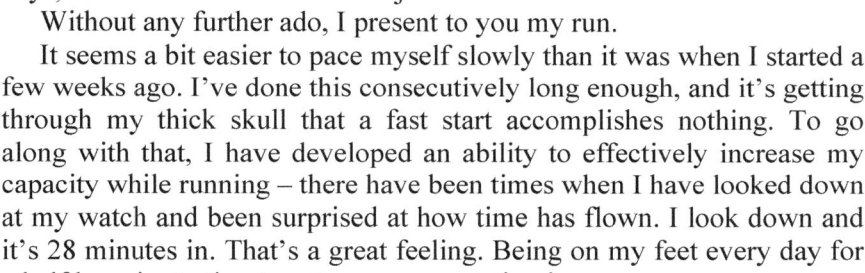

It's not cold, about 52 degrees. I should be nice and cozy from my body heat during the run.

The dread has abated today as I start my run – my soreness has lessened by this afternoon. Another few hours of rest and I bounce back?

Despite my series of "blech" days, I feel like I have a bit of mojo back.

Without any further ado, I present to you my run.

It seems a bit easier to pace myself slowly than it was when I started a few weeks ago. I've done this consecutively long enough, and it's getting through my thick skull that a fast start accomplishes nothing. To go along with that, I have developed an ability to effectively increase my capacity while running – there have been times when I have looked down at my watch and been surprised at how time has flown. I look down and it's 28 minutes in. That's a great feeling. Being on my feet every day for a half hour is starting to set a new expectation in me.

It's encouraging to me – and should be to you too – that a series of bad runs and increasing soreness is not necessarily followed by more bad runs and increasing soreness. At least at this distance, my body seems to have bounced back.

I have always had an appreciation for a complex problem – a problem without a clear, simple solution. A problem that requires consideration of other factors and requires you to weigh those factors against each other.

For example, I want my city, Mukilteo, to have more sidewalks. It would be more pedestrian-friendly. But sidewalks don't generate tax revenue. They might attract a certain type of population, and they can certainly have eye appeal in a residential community, but they don't generate money. In fact they require large sums to build and to maintain. So you have to weigh the pros and cons against each other. And while your gut instinct may be overwhelmingly "pro," you have to consider those "cons."

Running is similar. Whether or not I can grow to like it is similar. There are so many cons. So many moments of "ow this hurts," and "Why am I doing this?" and "who came up with this stupid idea?" They are balanced by those moments where you can work a problem out while running, or have those moments of lucidity, or are able to hold those uncertainties in your mind(John Keats). Everything else momentarily falls away and you can grasp the totality of a concept or idea like never before.

Of course it's silly to say that running is an evolutionary step backwards. On the surface, it doesn't appear to be forwards, really. I understand that's a debatable issue. But if running gives us those moments where we engage our creative selves in ways we never have before, then it may very well be forward. If man's ability to run allows him to maximize the use of his brain and solve more complex problems, you could make a counter argument that running is absolutely a step forward.

I think I just made a very convincing argument for talking Cheetahs. Since they don't exist, I am forced to reconsider my position.

Before you go to sleep, you can take advantage of your subconscious mind's ability to solve problems by considering a problem. As you sleep, your mind can creatively wrestle with the problem, and it might help you solve it. It's called "lucid dreaming," where you manipulate your dreams in the direction you want. Isn't this a bit like what we're trying to accomplish with running? Doesn't running give us those moments, and allow us a bit of silence to wrestle with our thoughts?

Fifteen minutes in and I lose steam again. This is getting old.

What I mean to say is that this performance level is getting old.

I can't argue with those wonderful moments I've had while running, I can't argue with the deconstruction of self. I do take umbrage at the fact that I am a slow ass old guy who is not improving. I always come back to that, some measure of the quality of a run, and whether or not I can like it. The quality of a run is measured by performance, in my mind.

Quality is by nature subjective. All of my pre-conceived notions with regard to running are subjected to my own quality measure. This moment, for instance, as I run along and consider my state, is a moment of import that I am able to get to while running. I can clear away the cobwebs sometimes and articulate things that can be difficult at other times. How do you measure that in terms of "quality?" How do you measure that in relation to other artificial quality measures, like whether you can grow to love something? Where's that metric?

The rain continues to drizzle down and my next thought is of how wet I'm going to be at the end of this run.

It's only now that I am fifteen minutes in; I was guessing before and I was wrong. I looked at my watch and expected it to be twenty minutes. I talked about being surprised at how far along I am. This time I'm surprised I'm not farther.

A run will always surprise you.

That could be what I learn to like about running. Whether it's a good surprise or a bad surprise, you'll always be surprised.

I think "if I could keep up this pace, I'd be okay! I'd be a ten minute mile runner." My wife hit that the other day. Good for her. And I suck.

Have you noticed? All of my words are formulas. All of my measurements are false. Running shatters my expectations. Every day.

It's as if I have been speaking the wrong language. I express everything as time over distance(pace). I expect everything to get better than it was. It's not just that everything isn't better than it was, it's that you should never expect things to be better than they are. You should expect them to be what they are, and find enjoyment in what is.

Running doesn't build you up – it just tears your body down. With it, you can remake yourself in whatever image you choose. You can't do that if you're like I am, always expecting it to be different, better. If you do, then practically every run is a failure by definition.

Look at me now, I'm the running philosopher. I wonder if Kant or Kierkegaard ever went jogging.

I round the corner, past the high school, elementary school, to the middle school. I'm pretty free this run, my motions feel natural and fluid. A tiny bit of foot pain, but not much to complain about this run. We're nearing Thanksgiving this month, and I have a lot to be thankful for, even in this run, don't I?

I pass the junior high and wave to a dozen kids there, who make fist-pumping motions. I think they are cheering me on! Either that, or they are jeering me on. I'm going with cheering.

I just discovered the etymology of "jeer." It's a "cheer" with a "joke." A joke-cheer. A portmanteau.

The wind picks up and the temperature drops a tiny bit as I round the corner to the YMCA. Yay hot tub. There are worse ways to end a run than in a hot tub!

My last thought for today strikes me as I hit the stopwatch at the entrance. Benjamin Franklin said that "Any fool can criticize, condemn, and complain - and most fools do." I've been a fool all my life. Sarcasm, the lowest form of wit, has been a close companion for many years. When I started this experiment, it was mostly with sarcasm. It hasn't served me well as I try to think objectively about running. It's been my greatest impediment. While there's no chance in Hades that I will suddenly go goody-two-shoes on life, I do need to recognize that there are some "pros" to running that I have been discounting in favor of the far more snarky "cons."

But the only one I am "conning" here is myself.

## Day 24 Results:
Weight: 243
Miles: 2.87 (watch)
TOF: 31 minutes, 00 seconds
10:48 average pace
Mood: Philosophical. (Freud says that I run because of my mom.)

## Pathetic Runners

I talked about my experience on one running forum, but I'm beginning to think that forum is the exception. Some running forums are a bit snobby, full of the arrogance of the youthful with a few oldsters chiming in with a more wizened grace. For the most part, runners are nice people. On the whole, I haven't really met many runners in person that I didn't think were good people. They are as nice as people who grow roses. As nice as people who love puppies.

Yesterday, I chanced upon a post on Facebook. It was regarding a runner, a mother, whose life was taken suddenly. She belonged to a group of runners called "pathetic runners group." With little more understanding than that, I sent in a request to join the group. I mean, Pathetic runners?

The group is moderated, in part, by runner and author David Johndrow. It's full of positive support for runners of any level, with much love for those of us who struggle. It sounds like a place we all are meant to be. It sounds like my running life. It sounds like family.

## 25. "YOU CAN MAKE IDEAS ...IN THE GARDEN OF YOUR MIND" – MR. ROGERS, MR. ROGER'S NEIGHBORHOOD

Our bi-weekly Costco trip was today. Only a few days before Thanksgiving, so we expected it to be ridiculously busy. What we got wasn't just crazy busy. It was just madness. It was mad, I tell you.

Pies. Around Thanksgiving, people make a decision to really like pies. Really like them. Everyone must have pie. They like pies enough to wait for them to come out of the bakery in the back of Costco and stack them in their cart like each of them is buying enough for their own pie-eating contest. They're playing ultimate Frisbees with their cart, trying to get as many points as they can.

Why would people practically crash into each other to get a pie? It's like Sharks hitting chum. It's a contact sport. We push our cart to the outside of the fracas, feeling like Roy Scheider in a boat catching a glimpse of something we can't believe we're seeing.

People walk in front of my wife, oblivious, as they remember something on their shopping list. They cut suddenly across the aisle. There's no "whoops, excuse me" – even worse, they don't even seem to acknowledge that they've cut off a *person*. It's like you're piece of a door frame or wall that they just have to get through or around, an inconvenient object passing through their awareness, their vague awareness. My wife becomes visibly agitated. How do you demand that people treat each other as people? I guess I could throw a tantrum, screaming "Pay attention to each other!" But the last time I did that it was amazing how fast those men showed up with the van and the gurney.

This is a public place, but I wonder if this how people act around their friends and loved ones at Thanksgiving? These people are shopping for their Thanksgiving feast – a day of Thanks. Will their Thanksgiving gathering be full of people as empty and clueless as they are today? Or is this the new "public" persona in society? Is Thanksgiving for them a sad play at life, a day of "sound and fury, signifying nothing"?

A Thanksgiving prayer: "I'd like to give thanks for the fact that my life was spared as I shopped for food this week, and I wasn't trampled."

We save the trampling for the day AFTER Thanksgiving, don't we.

A woman mutters to herself as she blocks an aisle. I stand right in front of her, expecting her to move, since her cart blocks my way to my left and she blocks straight ahead. She continues muttering, and finally steps back – not because she sees me, but because she wanted to look at something on the shelf above. I say "thank you" as I pass, but I'm not sure she saw me as I walked a foot in front of her eyes, or heard anything. This is probably the norm in most of her life.

A cashier politely asks if a woman might move her cart back so they can finish helping the person in front of her please? The woman can't even muster a grumble of consent: she just quietly rolls her cart back six inches, staring ahead silently, zombie-like.

When did we turn into automatons incapable of acknowledging each other?

Are society's collective meds so strong that we're reduced to a post-apocalyptic caricature of shopping zombies?

Black Friday is coming, and the brainless zombies shamble towards Wal-Mart: "Must… find…. Deals…"

But we survive our death by a thousand carts at Costco and head home.

On our way back from Costco, we come upon the scene of a one-car accident. A white Ford Thunderbird is half-off the median and into the other lane, with a broken axle. The right rear tire angles upwards like a real-life cartoon car from a Pixar movie.

As we pass, I mention to my wife that I should help. Two people sit in the car, but it's sitting in oncoming traffic in a busy intersection where two lanes turn directly into it. My wife does a quick U-Turn on the next street over; I get out of the car with my phone and go approach the couple. It's a young couple, twenties-ish, and they are just sitting in the car like they are in a parking lot, not sitting in a stationary car facing oncoming traffic.

"Are you okay?" I mouth to them as I approach the window.

"Yes," the girl in the passenger seat says, rolling the window down.

"Did you call 911?"

"We called Triple-A. They'll be here in two minutes."

"I'm just afraid someone will come around this corner and clip you."

"Well, they'll be here in two minutes."

146

"Two minutes," I repeat, importantly.

I go to the median where cars are turning and try to motion for oncoming traffic to slow down and move to the left. The couple sits in their car. Do they have a death wish? Is it fun to watch cars alternately step on the gas to zoom around their car, or brake suddenly to avoid hitting them? Get out of the car, morons. They remain in the car.

I try to direct traffic from the safety of the median, but at minute four I call 911. After a couple transfers(no one is hurt, after all), I end up at the Mukilteo dispatcher. The police are only a few minutes away. The tow truck arrives as I'm talking to the dispatcher. I have no idea if he can get a car with a broken axle onto his truck – it's not a hook truck, it's the flatbed variety.

I direct traffic until the police arrive. Still, people are idiots. A suburban locks up their wheels because they either don't know the sign for "slow down," don't care, or don't believe me. Another SUV almost merges directly into the engine block of an eighteen wheeler.

Once the police officer arrives, things settle down. People get a lot more cautious seeing flashing lights. I wait for a few minutes, then approach the officer, make sure the officer knows I called it in, didn't see it, and am leaving. I walk home, about a mile or so. I would turn this into my run and do another couple miles, but I don't have my futuristic recording device, so it becomes a reflective walk.

Isn't that just pathetic. I could have run, you see, but I wouldn't have been able to time it accurately or record my thoughts, so I walk home.

## "I don't care about any of you people"

What conclusion do I draw from this weird morning? I am witness today to that old saying "common sense ain't that common," but I'm also seeing so much oblivity.

Everything I've seen shocks me, because so many people aren't aware of what is happening at any given time. It's all about being present in the moment. Understanding what is happening to you right now. It's something we teach our kids when we teach them to cross the street. Situational awareness.

I have moments of oblivity, sure. I play video games. My wife can't even talk to me when I'm playing the banjo because my head is elsewhere, or when I am typing a letter to the editor, or my book, or Facebook.

But is this the new norm for our public moments now? When did being in public become a time for ignoring the rest of the public?

I believe ignorance like this probably started at about the time people started wearing pajama pants around town. That's the ultimate in "I don't care," isn't it? I don't expect anyone to walk around saying hello to perfect strangers, but pajama pants are an extreme response. Pajama pants say "If I knew any of you, I might put on a pair of pants. But truthfully, I don't care about *any of you people*."

It's a run right here in my neighborhood today after our strange Costco experience, after helping with an accident where people couldn't be bothered to get out of their car to save their life.

I'm going up the street, I'll take a left to about the halfway point and turn around. That's it. I'll go close to the scene of the earlier accident to where the Mukilteo community garden is. So I'll be running from the garden of my house, through the garden of my mind, to the Mukilteo Community Garden. And back.

It's a rainy, misty, foggy experience today. Still warm at 53 degrees. Normal November weather, a tiny bit warmer than usual. I wear my gloves because it's raining more than yesterday, as well as my light Brooks vest that I love so much; it's like a film that covers my torso.

This is one of those runs where you lace up not because you're excited about the day. You lace up because you want to be done. It's a day where I looked outside and said to myself "I want to be done with my run already." But wishful thinking doesn't make it so. Ughhhh. An obligatory run.

It's like taking out the trash. I have to go take out the trash, it will take me half an hour and I have to run there. It's time to do the chores.

Today the nike+ watch wins the satellite linkup competition – handily. The Forerunner can be persnickety, sometimes.

You'd think that after 24 days in a row of running I'd be prepared to make a decision, to call this thing already and state unequivocally that "I now forever despise running!" or "I am madly in love with running!" Nope. I'm still skeptical. I do think there is a value to doing this all at once, 30 days in a row, a trial by fire for running. But I'm not ready to "out" myself as either for or against running. What would my friends say if I outed myself like that?

As I discovered yesterday, the day before that and the day before that, my lack of joy for running might all be attributed to the garbage that I've lived with in my head for so long about expectations. I'm taking out the trash, all right. Taking out my mental trash.

I get to it.

I should make a little "plug" for Muscle Milk here. I used to drink it when I was working out more at the gym, and it was an incredible recovery drink for me. I've only had it twice in this experiment, just a scoop of powder in milk. It seemed to eliminate some soreness and help me recover both times. Back when I did more weight training, I could tell the difference after taking muscle milk and days when I didn't. It was a huge difference. Even experimenting with a couple of other recovery drinks I found that Muscle Milk worked better for me. Find whatever works for you.

The first mile of this run is uphill, so there is a good chance for me to have a negative split. I have a little bit of hip soreness on the right today which is accented on the uphill as I stretch my foot out farther with each step.

I take a walk break quickly today. Yipes, this is a tough hill.

I hit the bike path at .8 miles and glide effortlessly along, floating like a bird on wing.

Just kidding. This is work. Just work. The trick is enjoying the work in the garden of my mind.

Take heart, those who would be runners. If you keep doing this for long enough, you start fooling yourself into thinking you can do it. You can fake it till you make it. And who cares if you had to fake it if you make it? You're still making it! I start feeling good in this run, and I sense a source of power in my legs that I haven't felt before: the power that comes not from suddenly bounding along with a second wind, or from being able to run farther and faster. It's the strength that comes from ignoring pain. Knowing that you have pain and soreness but can run anyway. A kind of spiteful power.

I get to the fifteen minute mark, but I'm not to the Community Garden. It's about another quarter mile in. I push on, taking walk breaks when I need to. I'm trying not to get hung up on that stuff. A run is a run, even if it's a walk. It's my new definition.

I spend the middle of the run in a bit of a reverie thinking about recent events: the Ferguson, Missouri death of Michael Brown and the non-indictment of Darren Wilson by the Grand Jury. So much to unpack mentally in that situation, and I'm left thinking of all the nuanced arguments, and that it's a damned mess that exposes the worst in people.

Be better, people.

I stop at the Community Garden and take a quick break. Volunteers keep this going and their efforts result in dozens of pounds of food being donated every week to our Food Bank. A great way to make a difference in a community.

Is today promotion day? I'm plugging everything today. Well, what can I say? I'm motivated, I'm excited, having a good run, accomplishing a goal and feeling good about myself. I'm encouraged by the way that I'm achieving something I set out to do.

I have a big race before me on the 30th, let's not forget that. Mentally,

I feel like I've done some decent prep work.

It's always worse in your mind, isn't it? I expected to have stories about how my ankles were bleeding, how I shattered my spleen and had to be rushed to the hospital, how I was diagnosed with *delirium runnerensis*. My expectation was that at some point I might have to abort the mission. The reality of this experiment is that it is far easier than I thought it would be, at least from a physical perspective. It's the dread, the fear that you don't even feel, it's just there behind your actions, subtly driving them. The fear is always worse than the actual.

(Author's note: *delirium runnerensis*? That's not a real thing, but I have found that if you put something in italics and add "ensis,""atrophia," or some other latin-sounding suffix, you increase your credibility because it seems like a real thing. Don't show up at the doctor's office spouting nonsense because you read it in my book. I got enough problems of my own.)

I feel like this experience is burning the dross off of my thoughts and purifying them. My preconceptions, my expectations. It is tearing me down in a way. I wouldn't say it's changing me into something else, but I am a bit more humble in some ways and a bit more proud in some ways. I'm humbled by my continued failures in each run, and I'm a bit proud of the little things I'm accomplishing. The power of a goal, even a weak-seeming one, is that it can give you strength.

Hope. Why am I always so hopeful? Why, here at the mid-run point, do I suddenly rally and tell myself "here we go with the GOOD part of the run!" Why would the second half of the run be better than the first? I do this all the time. I'm so constantly optimistic. Why do I convince myself that everything is going to be better? And does talking to myself in this way take away from my ability to enjoy the moment? Why can't I enjoy right now RIGHT NOW, and worry about later, uh, later?

I feel my mechanics going to heck as I hit mile two. I try to focus on keeping my body upright to minimize strain on my back. On good "Chi."

Chi…Chai ..Tea Lattes. Man, remind me never to take up meditation.

Starting to feel a bit shin-splinty on the way down, but its 36 minutes in so I take a walk break. I might have to get rid of my unnatural fear of stretching to get rid of this feeling. I hear stretching can be good for you.

Why do I always have the feeling I am faster than I am? In my head I'm doing seven minute miles. I look at my watch. Ten minute miles, more like, when I'm not taking a walk break.

The rain comes down a bit harder, which has the effect of increasing the mist and restricting visibility to about a quarter-mile. I'm trotting it out downhill, which feels great.

I'm at the tail end of this thing, and feeling pretty good. You hear that world? I am feeling pretty good!

I am absolutely soaked, and loving the feeling of being in the moment.

## Day 25 Results:

Weight: 243
Miles: 3.43(nike+)
TOF: 40 minutes, 21 seconds
11:48 average pace
623 kcal
Mood: Kickin ass, actually.

## 26. "BE HERE. BE PRESENT. WHEREVER YOU ARE, BE THERE." – WILLIE NELSON

I am all the way down to 241 pounds today. I ate a carrot yesterday, so YEAH, killing it. I eat two more today to lock down my weight loss habit.

**My Best Words**

I know I'm not curing cancer with this experiment. I'm not trying to create a magical text of enchantment. I'm just documenting my sometimes pathetic thoughts. I'm not waiting for my best words. I'm writing the words I have to describe what I'm doing and feeling. It's not earth-shaking. It's important, perhaps, to no one but me. All stories are important to the owner first, but importance is a judgment each of us makes and places like a scarlet letter on things, a judgment that mirrors our own interpretation as much as it reflects reality. This story is important to me, and the words are only a vehicle to "out" the story. They aren't my best words, but they tell my story. They play my song. And as a lovely blogger I went to college with, Tina Kunz, said in her post today:

"Who needs to play the freshest instrument in the orchestra?"

It's just a work of love, running and writing about it. It marries two things that I have long been interested in. A marriage of convenience. An arranged marriage.

Will it last?

My wife asked me yesterday "how's it going?" Which seems like a really basic question, a simple question, but I didn't have a ready answer.

The only way I can describe how I'm feeling is that I am shaken by this experience. Not in an "I just saw the movie *The Shining* again. Hold me!" kind of way. More like the foundations of my beliefs are shaken. It feels precarious, like running is newer than it was a month ago, like I'm William Hurt in "Altered States" and I'm getting in touch with something deeper and more unpredictable in me.

At one point I felt like I was being pulled to a conclusion, one way or another. But now I feel more like my preconceptions have been stripped down and I am questioning whether or not I'll have a conclusion – or even that I *should* have a conclusion. Is conclusion the point?

So on the one hand this is a paltry little effort, running 30 minutes a day, a tiny thing that anyone can do. On the other hand, it's had an enormous effect on me. It's had an enormous effect on the way I perceive myself and the way I perceive running.

So I'm left holding the bag here. I set myself up for a grand conclusion on the last page, this incredible revelation, this internet meme of a moment, but I'm a little worried that when I get to unwrap that present, it might be empty.

And I'm feeling okay with that.

Running is a constant challenge. It's a puzzle. Is the joy of a puzzle finishing it? Of course not, the joy is in doing it.

We can be so un-self-aware sometimes. So unaware of who we are, how we are perceived. What we are about. And we ARE us, you know? So you'd think we'd have us figured out. In my case, I don't have me figured out.

I have an old bump on me from a surgery a half dozen years ago. It was the result of a lump I had under the armpit, which didn't show up on a scan, so the doctor recommended exploratory surgery. They found nothing, and as they sewed up the armpit they created a permanent lump. Isn't that clever of them? They figured out nothing and permanently created what they were trying to eliminate – a bump in my armpit.

Put another way, they examined a temporary lump and created a permanent bump.

Needless to say, I hate it, but I have grown used to it. Today I was putting on deodorant and was shocked to realize that it looked to be getting smaller. It's an armpit bump, and it's been the same since the surgery. No change, until today. I was genuinely surprised – this was totally unexpected.

So I asked my wife. "Honey, can I show you something weird?" And I took off my shirt.

"Oh my gosh, hon," she said, aghast, looking at the bump.

"Uh, what do you mean?" I was suddenly worried.

"I've never seen it look like that."

I brightened, "You mean this size?"

"Yeah, she said. I've never seen it so big."

Self-awareness? Not so much.

A few years prior, in a totally unrelated story, I visited my primary care physician when I neared forty years old, having the dreaded talk about what goes wrong as you get older. I really liked that physician because he answered practically everything I asked, and we talked about everything from hair loss to hemorrhoids to colonoscopies and prostate testing. It was actually just a checkup, and my tests looked good. I was fine, but I was so relieved and excited to have a physician so keen on answering all of my questions. Isn't it nice to discuss these things before they happen?

So the doctor gathered my file and went to the door. When he reached it, he turned around and said "So, if you want to do anything about that, now is the time."

I was puzzled. "Do I want to do anything about what?"

"Your hair loss."

"What hair loss?"

I really liked that Doctor and was sorry to see him go.

For a long-time, I considered myself self-aware. I'm sure you think that too. Guess what? I don't think I am anymore. I think I am ridiculously vain, ego-driven, and have been too stupid to realize it. Running has definitely made me confront that. Every DAY it makes me confront that. If you only run once or twice a week, you don't get that mojo going where you can fix your self-talk. When you run every day, you mind starts to show its colors and now you have to do something. When I was running once or twice a week, that's easy. I can be dishonest that often and it's okay. Forcing myself to run every day means that I have sniffed out my dishonesty. I am MacGruff the crime dog, a bloodhound, and I have smelled the B.O. of my vanity and found it most foul. I shall chase it into the shadows.

By running it away?

I remember that on my very first run, down into the Bob Hierman Wildlife area in Snohomish, I thought about how running is primal and we use it to run to something or away from something. I never, ever thought that what I might be referring to was running to and away from yourself. But that seems pretty evident to me now. I was running from *me*. In running more often, I am starting to find a way to run back to *me*.

I'm keeping with the theme of challenging myself today and going back to my hardest course, which is Japanese Gulch. It's crazy hilly, difficult to navigate, so I'm going to plug away at it and continuously improve myself.

Nike+ watch lovers, I'm abandoning you. It's not you, it's me. Don't let this come between us. This watch won't sync anymore, and I have no patience for things that won't sync with my life, you know? It is the digital age, and this watch isn't keeping up with the times.

I was thinking it might be colder here, closer to Puget Sound, but it's fantastic. Slightly overcast, a tiny bit of sun, no rain and somewhere over fifty degrees with no wind. It's a great day to run. It's tough to run at a constant cadence up hill, so I just put on some regular old bluegrass and rock and roll for today.

I do my funny dance of starting one watch, then starting the other watch, then looking back to make sure the first watch is running, then looking at the second watch to make sure my second watch is running, then covering up the first watch with my sleeve, then covering the second watch with my sleeve. Dear reader: abandon watches. They are so lame. Makes me want to run without watches. Or without my music too, why not. Also a shirt. Do I really need shoes? Look, I've discovered streaking. I've also discovered my next book's cover image.

It's a muddy trail – if there is a run I am going to fall, this is it. I'm not including the half-marathon, which will probably include a faceplant. I wind up switchbacks, up the side of the gulch. The tough part of Japanese Gulch, in addition to the elevation gain, is that there are so many crisscrossing trails. I try to make a series of right turns so I can find my way back if I need to without calling in air transport.

I reach the top of the trail and think about the idea of running by yourself. It is different than running with someone. It is for yourself, and no one else. There's Ralph Waldo in my mind again: "Every man alone is sincere. At the entrance of a second person, hypocrisy begins"

The top of Japanese Gulch has a plateau on one side with a more open forest. My series of right turns takes me to the outer perimeter of the park, a bit of a plateau. It's already been twelve minutes and I'm barely at the top of the Gulch. Japanese Gulch is wider than it is long, and I've basically run the width of the trail. The length of it stretches off through the trees. I focus on working on form, stride, and on not slipping.

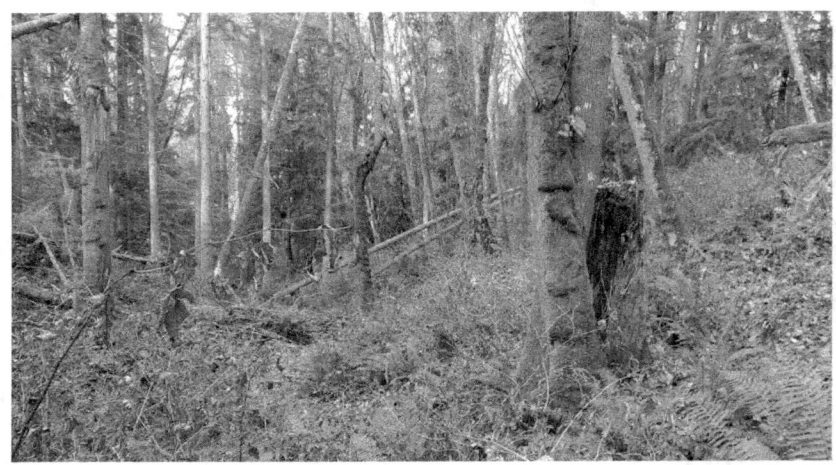

My watch is not picking up my progress again – too many switchbacks. It says .8 miles in fifteen minutes. Gah. Japanese Gulch is a windy enough trail that I can't really focus on whether or not my watch is performing; I can only focus on myself. That and making sure I can find my way out of here.

I think of performance. My watch's measure of my time is an artificial measurement that only has meaning in relation to something else. Miles per hour, total miles, some artificial "point" that we have decided is our raison d'etre, but which is really external to running itself. Running is just running. We attach meaning, "good," or "bad," and if we do so based on relative, arbitrary measures then we run the risk of making it less meaningful. Especially if we are running for fun. What does the passage of time have to do with running in its purest form? If we are running specifically to improve our time, of course that is different. If we are running to run greater distances, that's different. If we are running for exercise, fun, motivation, then measuring our performance according to time and distance is ridiculous. It's as ridiculous as measuring how much fun a child is having by the amount of time they play with one toy.

Similarly, our whole concept of "performance" is rooted in the idea of artifice. Actors perform, which is to say they act like someone else, something external. We judge them as "good" or "bad" based on our judgment of how well they pretended to be something they are not. Isn't that an odd way to measure anything? Don't get me wrong. I love me some Breaking Bad. Heisenberg really was "the one who knocks." Cranston was spectacular in that show, but we judged his performance because it was so *believable* – not real, but *believable*. As in, "I was able to believe it." That word contains the idea that it's not real. Running isn't about lifting weights at the gym, looking at yourself in the mirror and trying to make yourself into something you're not. Running is just you. Just you. That's real as it gets.

So if I'm saying I am performing well on my run, I'm really saying that I am doing something artificial. How was your run? Good! Bad! Those words should be enough, though they don't capture the whole experience, to be certain. We should stop concerning ourselves with outcomes and excluding our perception of the moment in any way we can. Stop pretending to be something we're not. Just enjoy the moment – or if the moment is terrible, that's okay too. Life has terrible moments. Like when your Doctor says you have a receding hairline and you were too dense to realize it.

I wrote papers in college where the whole goal was to draw conclusions. To take the information you were given and discern meaning. This experiment, which was designed to get me to one of two possible conclusions, has made me question the question. Why am I so eager to draw conclusions? Like a stopwatch, how is that not an artificial measure?

I turn back, almost unintentionally, down another intersecting trail that takes me straight back to the edge of the Gulch, where more switchbacks immediately take me down. That was fortuitous.

I run next to the treetops to my right, lower than me as the gulch descends. I loop down quickly to the path I started on. It's not about speed here, because the footing is just as difficult going down as it was coming up.

So I think I've been letting the good be the enemy of the great. I am absolutely guilty in my life of striving to make things perfect, and not completing things because, in my opinion, they weren't ready. With a bit more work, they really were ready. I have let my desire for greatness stop me from doing good work.

Good is enough for practically everything. This is a good run. Not a perfect run, but a good run. I finish strong back to the parking lot.

## Day 26 Results:
Weight: 241
Miles: 1.71??
TOF: 31 minutes, 01 seconds
Hahahaha: average pace
Mood: The journey is the goal.

## 27. "THE SECRET OF CHANGE IS TO FOCUS ALL OF YOUR ENERGY, NOT ON FIGHTING THE OLD, BUT ON BUILDING THE NEW" – SOCRATES

"I suck at this," Says my nine-year old.

It's Thanksgiving, and we're shucking the papery skin off of cloves of garlic. He separates all the cloves but leaves the harder inside layer on. He makes his announcement re suckage and abruptly quits to go play Minecraft. I let him know later he should practice this skill in Minecraft so he gets better at it. I'm not sure he gets the sarcasm.

Shucking garlic is actually something he's surprisingly good at. We've done it before when we were on a garlic kick, when we went through a clove or two a day with different recipes. He got very good at it.

But he's nine, so that doesn't matter. For all I know he does know he's good at it, but just wants to be off-duty.

Also, I wonder where he would ever develop a thought process like "I suck at this?"

Yeah, I'm guilty as charged. I don't walk around saying "I suck at this" ever, but I do say things periodically like "I hate running." I don't perceive that as melodramatic. Obviously, as previously noted, my self-perception is off. I'm not special.

YOU'RE NOT SPECIAL
YOU'RE NOT "AWAKE"
YOU'RE NOT ENLIGHTENED
YOU'RE NOT ONE OF THE FEW
YOU'RE NOT AN EXPERT
YOU'RE NOT AN INVESTIGATOR
YOU JUST HAVE INTERNET
ACCESS

I have worked at fighting the old for 27 days. Now it's time to build the new.

A family run today, to celebrate Thanksgiving. Our own little turkey trot. Why not? We're about to celebrate the pilgrim's desire to overeat in a few hours, so we might as well try to run that off in advance.

We'll run Big Gulch. We wish our neighbors a happy Thanksgiving, get a picture. I give the children key instructions about staying together through certain parts of the run near the street, and we're off.

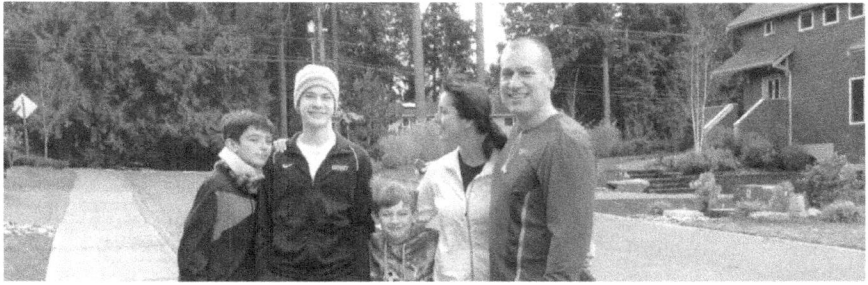

A little mist falls upon us and the crowd goes wild – my kids squeal with delight. Weirdos.

As we crest the hill, we see additional rain off in the distance across the water. We might get wetter.

My twelve-year old likes to take off in the lead, but he has developed a false sense of security. During cross country team's practice he runs on a part of the street with no sidewalks, and I fear that has given him the bad habit of not watching what cars are doing and assuming that they will always behave. On our last turn before we descend into the gulch proper, he takes the turn, near an overhanging bush, without consideration of the fact that a car might be coming. This isn't a busy area and I doubt there are more than a dozen cars that roll along this street per day, but I can't avoid a parent heart-attack moment. "We need to stay together!"

I give the kids another stern Daddy warning about what to expect during the next section of the run. I tell the boys they can "turn it loose" in the gulch a bit, once we arrive, speedsters. Once we get there. In the meantime you have to be slow like Dad.

We run to the bottom of the hill, still a bit ahead of Mom. We run past a City Council member in Mukilteo walking his dogs. We wish him a Happy Thanksgiving.

The boys run ahead up the hill to the gulch "proper," and I wait at the bottom for Denise. She's less than 30 seconds behind me. I start up the hill, and find myself taking walk breaks on each switchback series, but I still feel strong and steady.

Now that I'm not concerned with child safety, let's see how I do!

At the midpoint, I realize that I haven't looked at my watch once to check my time. Am I finally breaking the habit? Mayyybe.

I stop to make sure a well-mannered Labrador doesn't make a sudden move towards my wife. I say well-mannered because the owner has him sit off to the side of the trail obediently. He's a portly old dog and has a red bandana around his neck. Has anyone ever been attacked by an old fat lab wearing a bandana? Seems unlikely.

I know that stopping means that my wife will probably catch up and take the lead. Thinking about performance, suddenly. Hello old friend. At least I'm conscious of it.

Socrates mentioned "building the new." It's difficult to develop new habits out of thin air. Force of habit and old expectations come back if they are not displaced by new thought patterns. This is a problem I have unwittingly built into my experiment. I've tried to have no expectations, but I thought falsely that I was a "clean slate" coming in. Obviously I was not. The way I have approached running for so long poisons me at every step, and rushes in even when I push back, a wall of water that flows through my mental fingers.

It's like being a parent. We might agree or disagree with what our parents did, but when we have children ourselves, we default to the only style we know – our parents' style.

So now I'm caught in a bit of a conundrum. If I focus on performance, on pace and time, that gives me something to aim for, but it doesn't capture what I'm looking for – the *quality* of a good run. Whatever that means.

A "tinybuddha" article that says this: "If you want to experience more love, start giving more love." Can I apply this to running? Does that mean that I should run more if I want to enjoy it more? Good news, I'm doing it. I can't help but feel I am on the right track to looking beyond my own distractions. "Building the new" is about creating new ideas about running. I take that as meaning: I need to read more about other runners, other successes and other failures. Think more about mechanics, form and what makes a "quality" run.

I even have to decide what "good" means for me. What is a good run? At a really strange level I feel like Bill Clinton explaining himself during the Monica Lewinsky scandal. Famously, he clarified what "is" means in front of a grand jury.

As I wrestle with myself, my wife passes me.

So what makes it a good run? I could argue that every single run is a good run. I've challenged myself physically. I've challenged myself mentally. I've had moments of clarity and an explosion of ideas at certain times. The journey is the destination. I'm not sure I ever understood that before. It's remarkably difficult to be present in every moment. We tend to think of the next moment. And past moments.

That's what our watch is: a log of our past moments. "Past performance is no guarantee of future results."

We have legends about change, stories we hold dear. Examples of someone making a break with what they've done, changing on the inside and making changes in their life. That's what *A Christmas Carol* is. I am the Ebenezer Scrooge of running, possessing great wealth but hoarding it. And if you keep it inside, it means nothing. Scrooge changed his mind and life. He was "shaken," too, by spirits who showed him context in his life. How much easier has this challenge been? I didn't even have to see my death. It's a crucible of my own creation, but it appears to be having the same effect.

I pass my wife.

I pass my kids.

Performance! Yeah, but it feels good.

Of course, the kids catch up. I'm not Superman.

My youngest son tells me what he wants to do on a videogame when we get home. My new zen self loses its temper. Why do we want to talk about a video game when we are out here experiencing nature and running? Why is it so hard to be HERE?

What follows is a primer for my children on meditation. Like I'm suddenly an expert on that. Well, I try to be humble in my explanation, but I recognize that it's a ridiculous thing to try to explain what little I know of Buddhism to tiny humans who are thinking about what to do when they get home. It's ridiculous to explain to someone who is living for the next moment that they should be living in this moment, isn't it? It's like another language. An old man talking about the way things were when he was young strikes us as old-fashioned, too absorbed in history.

I must sound similarly anachronistic to my children, who talk about the future of their video game while I am "stuck" in the present. Anyway, as should be obvious by now, I fail miserably at the lesson.

As we get to the stairs, my youngest interrupts my lesson on meditation:

"They should make an escalator instead of stairs here."

Yes, he believes there should be an escalator in the middle of our trail run.

I get back to frustration at the end of the run – the kids bolt ahead and aren't looking around as they pass blind driveways, so the last half-mile is punctuated by me trying to yell ahead for them to look around. As we come into the house, I let them know why this is important.

Being present is all well and good, but you have to be safe. Suddenly, I am make an awkward full circle in my own rhetoric, talking about being present in the moment and telling kids who were talking of the future that they should indeed think of their future – because that's what looking around for cars is, thinking about the future. Parenting is a study in hypocrisy.

I'm not sure I built much new, but our family made some memories together, and we had fun, despite my anxiety. Looking forward or looking back can't always be a bad thing, can it? Is there a way to stay in the moment but still be aware of important things that happen around you, that have implications that you can react to – like an oncoming car?

I'm thankful. I'm thankful to be alive. I'm thankful to have learned so much this month about myself. I'm thankful to be nearly done with one of the most significant things I've ever done. I'm thankful for my family and friends.

After we eat, I calculate the amount of running I need to burn off the calories this Thanksgiving. So many zeros. I am getting confused by scientific notation. Is this amount measured in light-years?!?

## Day 27 Results: "Crowd Goes Wild"

Weight: 241
Miles: 2.71
TOF: 34 minutes, 36 seconds
12:42 average pace
Mood: Still exploring and enjoying the journey(when I'm not trying to keep my kids from getting injured).

## Flexibility

You know me by now. I want instant gratification. Total reward without the effort. It's the American Way, dangit.

In college I took a dance class. The guy with no flexibility. The guy who never took a dance class before. Now he's going to learn ballet. It was from someone with incredible dance experience and huge street cred, Idalee Hutson Fish. I was, as almost literally as I can describe it, a bull in a china shop.

I was in a dance show that semester, with all the waify women who gracefully stayed en pointe. I was straight out of Army training, so I looked good. A shirtless affair with Army BDU pants on. I think it was a vaguely abusive scene actually.

Like so many things, I didn't have the patience for flexibility. I had acting instructors who led us through all the normal body-loosening exercises, which seemed like so much claptrap. I'm sure they helped despite my reservations and cynicism. I'm sure I was a better performer because of it. I'm also sure I didn't get it.

I am not sure we needed so much flexibility in our youth, but as we age "stretch before and after workouts" sounds like really good advice. Don't stretch and you get sore, or injured. All around me people friends are popping their Achilles tendons, spraining groins, having stress fractures. We get old, man. Stretching is important.

I'm a big believer – TODAY- in stretching as a way to prevent soreness and cramping. I wish I would have believed in it years ago.

## 28. "LOSING AN ILLUSION MAKES YOU WISER THAN FINDING A TRUTH." – LUDWIG BORNE

I am so close I can taste it. Today, tomorrow, and Sunday. Right now I want to take off, get out the door early and get one step closer to completion. I had a crazy thought I would leave earlier, before eight in the morning, but the rain was coming down and I tasted the comfort of coffee.

It's only 42 degrees, but the wind and the cool rain makes it seem more like 42 kelvin. That's -384 Kelvin for you non-nerds. It's not funny if I have to explain it.

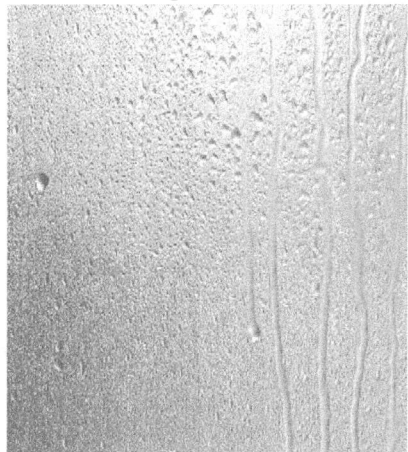

The rain doesn't relent. In fact, it might be raining harder. There is a possibility of snow later in the day, so that's another motivator. Tomorrow's run and the half-marathon might indeed suck – I'm talking empirically now, not subjectively – so if I can get today under my belt I'm one step closer.

I have little confidence in my watches in this weather. The Forerunner has been good lately, but it's tough to sync up with heavy cloud cover like this. Lo and behold the underdog nike+ syncs up perfectly. I could just use a stopwatch now and mapmyrun to figure out the distance, but obviously my nike+ watch wants back in my good graces.

I'm in full regalia today. Rain slicker, gloves, a hat. One of my main concerns is the wet. If I get my running shoes too wet, they may not dry out in time for Sunday. I'll give them a break tomorrow if it's still raining and use my old running shoes. It's these silly things you start to think about as a race looms. I hear that real runners put out their race outfits the night before, which I'm not sure is due to their desire to plan. More like fear. Fear that they will wake up early, get to the starting line, and realize they have forgotten something. On a cold wet day forgetting something can make a rough run all the more miserable. All of this preparation done for the sake of the privilege of moving your legs back and forth.

Have you ever decided to start doing something, you got ready to do it, and then suddenly you didn't want to do it? I'm like a capricious kid as I look outside my garage into this wet, wet day. Where is the Cat in the Hat when you need him.

It's wet enough that I'm concerned about my Futuristic Recording Device(FRD) today. I wrap it in a plastic grocery bag to protect the microphone from the rain. Classy.

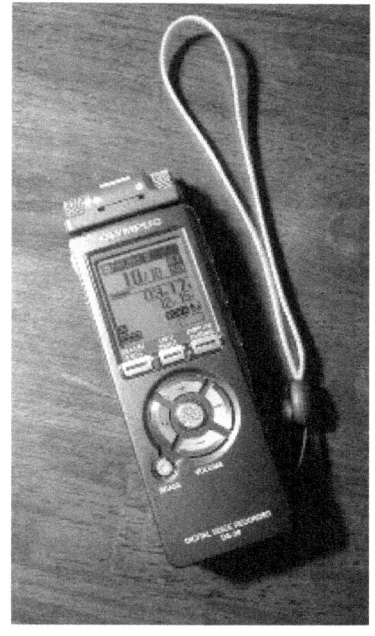

There aren't many cars on the road today as I start around my neighborhood, back up to the Mukilteo garden and back. All the Black Friday shoppers are out hustling goods away from other customers in the name of bargain-hunting. Everyone else is wisely at home.

I take my eye off the path and get a splat in the face from a rain-heavy branch. Ploosh!

Rivulets of rainwater flow across the sidewalk. Nature has thrown down the gauntlet and I am up to the challenge! Hills.

A long light at the top of the first hill, but I am glad for the respite. A sign of things to come: my fingers are already a little numb despite the light gloves.

A cooling greyish rain.

I hit the top of the hill, slowly. Instead of being a welcoming rest, the flatter part of the run is the windiest. The rain blows harder, pelts my eyes. I focus on form, elbows back, focus on the tip of the pendulum, legs kick to the rear.

Abruptly, I think "why did I not even consider the treadmill?"

Here's a tip: there's no comparison. My wife left this morning and went for a walk with her friends. She's in this icky weather too, and there is no comparison between running outside, or even being outside and running on a "dreadmill." Treadmills were invented by sadists who looked at running and wanted to duplicate the activity but squeeze any potential for enjoyment out of it. Running outside is to running on a treadmill what playing a boardgame is to reading the dictionary.

I take my mind off the course long enough to step in a puddle and soak my foot. Outstanding. So I favor the other foot long enough to step in another puddle with my other foot. A lovely wetness creeps into my shoes. Fan-Damn-tastic.

The puddles continue near the top of my turnaround point, so it's a series of leaps and bounds as I avoid them. I consider turning around before I get to the turnaround point at the garden – I'll still hit 30 minutes – but what point would that serve? It's not like I'll be any drier for it. So I continue along.

## Lessons from the Matrix

If my series of tactical lessons from this experiment begins with 1) don't wear a watch, then it continues with 2) run in inclement weather. I find myself out here not caring if I walk. I'm doing this. Just as taking away the watch takes away the pressure, running when it is super-crappy out also takes away pressure, so you can focus on running and finishing to the exclusion of everything else. Everything except rain pelting you in the face.

What are rules but things we break? I look at my watch at the turnaround point and realize I am molasses-slow. 22:00 for around 1.6 miles. I shouldn't have looked.

Strategic lessons: patience. It's a lesson I've tried to learn throughout my life. I've never been patient. I may seem patient, but I'm not. I'm practically mercuric in my mindset. I want to *do* it *finish* it be *done* RIGHT NOW. Over this last year, this last month I've realized how foolish that has made me. It's the matrix and I'm enamored with the woman in red, but miss the bigger point – the agent behind her. Not that it matters, for the whole thing is an illusion. There is no spoon. I was concerned with things that hardly matter in the first place.

The rain abates slightly.

The good news about running in the cold rain is that it's difficult to distinguish between soreness and being numb. I feel something, but I'm not sure what it is. Of course it doesn't matter. I have to ignore it anyway. I'm back in the matrix, rising above the reality, believing it isn't real.

Has anyone else noticed that you don't get better running the same distance? That a run doesn't really get "easier and easier?" I have been running roughly the same distance each day and showing no improvement in my physical ability. That is absolutely terrible – and I'm speaking qualitatively too. I had a moment at mile two where I thought "oh, yay, this is a nice easy part of the run" and a minute later it turns to "I am done with this!" Where is the "better" part?

A couple of crows pass overhead and land on a nearby yard, both carrying pieces of what appear to be dinner rolls. It's nice to see nature enjoying Thanksgiving leftovers too.

I continue to throw my body upon this pre-determined course, knowing this is just a terrible pace. The pace is not something I'm focused on, but it's still there. That's an interesting feeling, an innate conflict in my mind. Pace versus enjoyment. Lawful Evil versus True Neutral, for you Advanced Dungeons & Dragons runners out there. I know that's a large segment of the population.

A twinge in my ankle presents itself on the downhill. I hope it doesn't turn into something before Sunday. That leads to thoughts of how unprepared I am for the half-marathon. You'll recall my story of woe from my first half marathon years ago. Now I've decided to do it again as a kind of culminating project for this experiment, my Master's thesis on running badly. So I prepare for it by running every day, about one-quarter of the distance. How the heck does that work? Why in God's name would I expect this to be anything but an unmitigated disaster? So it seems like I am setting myself up to bomb. On the other hand, if I'm going to burn this running bug out of me, that might be the best way. Running is a fever that I am burning out of my body by wrapping myself tightly in blankets, daring the illness and sweating it out.

My feet are sore. I have to pee. My ankles are stiff as I run/walk the last quarter-mile. While I can claim victory with my time-on-feet today, I can't claim much more than that. It's another victory in my head, a moral victory. Turns out I was not really as up to the "challenge" today as I thought I was.

## Day 28 Results:
Weight: 241
Miles: 3.53
TOF: 44 minutes, 34 seconds
12:38 average pace
Mood: I'm ready! I'm not ready.

# 29. "LEAVE YOUR SITUATIONS AT THE DOOR." - MARY J. BLIGE

Snow! The day before I finish and there's a blanket of warm snow on the ground.

Okay, it's not exactly warm. It feels like Christmas out here.

I'm brushing snow off my car. The snow is melting slightly as the temperature hovers around freezing. A gorgeous beautiful day. Looks like it will clear up, but this will be a good training ground in miniature for the half marathon tomorrow.

Honestly, my biggest concern right now is finishing half marathon. Oddly, my second biggest concern is what to wear. There are chafing issues, you see. I've had chafing issues before and it is absolutely excruciating. Commando, or no? I'd like to not repeat the chafing situation, thank you sir.

Also - keeping warm is a concern! It's supposed to be twenty degrees tomorrow. Not only are we running thirteen miles(my wife and I, she is doing it too!) in below freezing temperatures; we're going to have to stand around for a bit at the starting queue.

So how do I keep warm before and during the race?

Yes, I'm thinking about clothes. And I will probably, yes, set my clothes aside for tomorrow, like a real running geek. That will make feel like a real runner – fake it till you make it - and it will help me keep from forgetting something. It will also take my mind off of potential disaster. Did I mention I'm running thirteen miles? That's 52 laps around a high school track. Ugh. If I started running from my house and ran that distance, I would get to north Seattle.

The temperature is beginning to drop already. It's the kind of snow that is not a problem once you get out of your unplowed neighborhood, but it could get worse by freezing any minute.

As beautiful as it looks outside with fresh snow on the branches, I've chosen to run at the industrial park near my house.

For one reason.

DONUTS!

Henry's donuts is the starting and stopping place for my run, and on a day where the temperature is 29 and there is fresh snow on the ground, I need all the inspiration I can get. That's my reward for myself on this day, one day away from completion. Sometimes you have to build those rewards in – and today I'll actually have that reward, unlike my previous psych-out of myself. Call it carb-loading, call it whatever you want.

Is it odd that on the second-to-last day I have to trick myself into running with a donut? It seems odd. And yet I donut care.

Today I am all about the plastic. I've got some things I am thinking about running in tomorrow, but today I'm wearing different clothes and layers of plastic. There is a plastic bag on my torso as a mid-layer between a long-sleeve technical shirt below and a short-sleeve technical shirt above it. I'm running with plastic gloves too – those nitrile gloves you get at Harbor Freight for staining bookcases. I hope they work to reflect my hands' heat back inward. The gloves will either be a complete failure or the best thing I have ever discovered. I'll be the guy running with blue gloves.

After I pull into the parking lot at Henry's, My nike+ watch links with the satellite immediately. Hoping for a good performance review at the end of the year? And in all fairness to the nike+, the Forerunner struggles again. It connects well, but then gives me a batteries low signal. That was the reason we stopped using that watch all the time – inconsistent performance. A theme for GPS watches.

As I leave Henry's and crunch across the new layer of snow, I think "it's about time for me to wrap this thing up. It's about time for me to start talking about what running means to me." With like, conclusions and stuff like that. It's been 29 days. Isn't that about enough? Yeah, I feel like it should be too.

It's not exactly easy to run along a sidewalk when the snowplow has been through and lifted the street snow up to the sidewalk level. The soft layer of snow is marred by a slushy top. Instead of running on a thin layer of vanilla frozen yogurt, I'm running on a thicker layer of chocolate chip mint. I know that sounds delicious, but I'd prefer vanilla at this point. Worst analogy ever.

Early on I'm cold, so that means I have to use speed to warm myself up.

A lot of calf soreness last night in bed. I tried using my wife's roller doohickey to self-massage them. Wow, that hurt like heck.

Part of my difficulty in concluding is that running is an experience. It's a different experience every time. So how do you draw conclusions when it's different every time? The only thing you can conclude is whether or not you like having different experiences all the time. And you know what? I do. I do like the adventure, either way, good or bad, even if the experience is hard to anticipate. That certainly keeps it interesting.

When I used to go to the gym, I'd have good days and bad days. A good day meant you lifted more. A bad day, you lifted less. But you could regulate that yourself and give yourself a break when necessary. Running isn't so forgiving. It's relentless. It doesn't ease up because you're having a bad day. The good news is that it doesn't really get harder either, even if it feels harder. Distance is a constant variable – it's you that is different. You experience the same thing differently, but running pushes it on you regardless of your ability to handle it. Running is fair. It may seem hurtful, but it is equitable in its distribution of punishment.

In an interesting way, running is an acknowledgement of how small you are – how *little* you are capable of. That makes the highs higher, because the lows are lower. When it sucks, It's hellish. But when it's good, it's glorious.

I've only seen a dozen or so cars on the streets here, but they each car has one thing in common: the drivers all look at me like I am crazy.

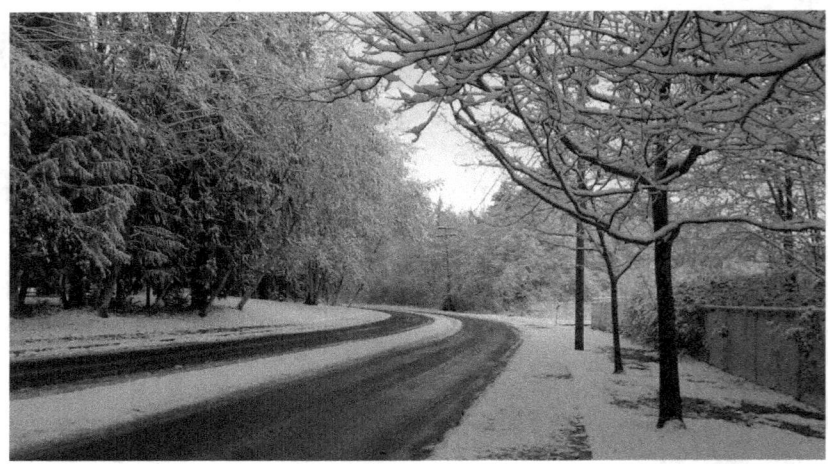

Plastics situation report(sitrep): Torso warmth holding stable. Nitrile gloves failing to maintain hand temperature. Recommend usage only with additional glove layer.

The crunchy layers of snow are a welcome cushion compared to running on a bike path, sidewalk, or trail. It's better than running on a beach because the snow is so much lighter, you can plow through it. It's like resting my feet today. Of course, we're only talking about an inch of snow here.

I'm only ten minutes in, but the first mile was a 9:00 pace. I allow a little self-congratulation. I slow down slightly and hope that doesn't cause me to get colder.

I think there is something wrong with the way I breathe. Not in a "call 911!" way, but in an "I burp a lot" way. I am probably gulping air. If, unlike me, you really take time to read through the literature, there is a tremendous amount to focus on. It's like working on your golf swing – it's always something, whether it's breathing from your diaphragm, the tilt of your hips, keeping the bottom half of your legs loose. There are always things to run down in your mental checklist.

The slipperiest part of the run is by the Fire Station, where some conscientious firefighter has been outside and shoveled a snow-shovel-blade width of snow away. The layer underneath has frozen to a slippery sheen.

By the halfway point in today's run, the wind has died down slightly and I'm warmer, even to my fingers. Tomorrow this will only equal a tenth of the distance. Yaaaaaay.

Like most days, running in inclement weather is a fine line between overheating and keeping your body warm enough. It's self-regulation. That is exactly what running is, regulating yourself. Keeping yourself regular. That's pretty funny if you go through the entirety of that double entendre.

It's self-regulation. Running lets you experience highs and lows so you can find your own middle. It's Boot Camp, where they break you down to build you up. When I was in Boot Camp, on day ONE the Drill Sergeants lined us up and started barking commands. They yelled at me for absolutely nothing. I didn't get my socks out of my rucksack on time, I was moving too slow, why didn't I have my canteen out already? I wasn't doing pushups fast enough. Of course it was entirely intentional. I finally broke down and cried. One of the things I have a problem with is being blamed for something I didn't think was my fault. It's a flaw I discovered early on.

My biggest lesson from Boot Camp: no matter how much yelling someone does, you can only do so many pushups before your arms fail. No matter how upset someone is, there is only so much you can do. It is a kind of mental touchstone. Your best is your best, and whether it's good or bad, it's all you have.

So this experiment, similarly, helps me find my center. This time, with less crying.

We don't think about these things as adults: how can we make sense of ourselves? At the risk of sounding hokey, that's a lot of what I've been working out.

"Do you like running Tony? Do you love it?"

Well, do you like getting presents?

"Of course I do. I love getting presents!"

What if you could get a present every day?

"That would be awesome!"

What if some of them were crappy presents? What if some days your present was a candy cane wrapped in horse manure? Would you still want to get presents every day?

I would.

I don't think this analogy is too far off. Running is a series of gifts that you give yourself, and some of them are terrible. Sometimes the places you go are awful, mentally. Sometimes the things you think and believe are great. It is up to you how you thread those things together, to make meaning of rats running across the trail, or to leave them as meaningless. To enjoy it for yourself or derive meaning. Some things don't have a discernable meaning. What then?

Running helps you train yourself to do the work and stop being invested in the result. It gets you out of the "instant gratification" mode, because on some runs there is no gift. Or it's poo. On some days, your gift is poo.

And then comes a new day. You have to let the horse manure days go. That's a simple life lesson that running makes you confront constantly.

Other days, the gift is rainbows. What I thought would be a pot of gold at the end of the rainbow may only be a tale whispered to me by my own leprechauns. I might get there and only see the end of the rainbow. Would that be so bad? I did see a rainbow for the entire time. Okay, some of the time, but that might be because I have a habit of taking my eye off the rainbow.

I may not be faster, but I have reset my expectations of running. Sometimes, running feels easy. I know that seems crazy to say. More accurately, the action, the motion of running fits with my mindset and allows my mind to alternately clear and fill. It's almost a mental "fasting" and purging.

Oh, and I take back everything I said about Chris McCandless being stupid. Sometimes in life you have to do something stupid to prove what you can do. My experiment is way down on the stupid scale, but I get that McCandless was a guy that wanted to do something different, audacious. Under a different set of circumstances, it might have worked out. Sometimes we can be too stupid. It doesn't make our audacity wrong.

I don't want this experiment to end with some kind of giant apology to the world... but if the running shoe fits. Strangely, I can't say I love running, but I am starting to develop an appreciation for it. It helps me turn things over in my mind, gives me a sense of peace - when it's not completely sucking.

That, incidentally, is the reason this is so hard to sort through. Its one thing to have gently conflicting thoughts in your head, but it's another thing to reach completely opposite conclusions based on nothing more than the moment you happen to be thinking about the problem.

Now it's time for a donut.

## Day 29 Results: "Way to Go"
Weight: 243
Miles: 2.78
TOF: 32 minutes, 11 seconds
11:33 average pace
Mood: Just another run in the snow. As you do.

## Saying "Hi" to Dean Karnazes

Packet pickup. My wife and I drive to Seattle to pick up our numbers and free shirt – a ritual I've done with her a dozen times. The slush has frozen in our neighborhood and it's a dicey proposition to drive up a couple of minor inclines. But I-5 is clear and we make it to the Westin. We valet park not because we're rich, but lazy. And we do the usual looking around at the Expo for stuff. I try on a pair of Hoka shoes, which feel like walking on a puff of air, but I don't buy any. I might sometime, but of course no WAY I'm throwing anything different in the mix for tomorrow. That's a cardinal sin.

My wife buys some merino wool socks for the race, and we head into a nearby conference room to see Dean Karnazes address the crowd.

Of course I thought he'd be taller. My wife says the same thing.

Dean has a bit of a pre-packaged talk where he talks about why he runs, how he does it, and what he eats. A small segment of talk punctuated by a video from letterman, his appearance on a Stan Lee shoe about being superhuman, or on the today show. He's done amazing, wonderful things, and despite his desire to appear self-conscious, it's obvious that he enjoys being a showman and in the spotlight. That's okay by me – he's done amazing things, and he should be proud.

He talks about being motivated to run extreme distances in extreme conditions, having completed a World Record 262 mile run and setting his eyes on 300. He's a bit of a motivational speaker as he talks of never giving up, of sacrifice and training. Hallucinations, passing out, running a nine-hour marathon in the South Pole, and training by running through the night…!

Dean said in an almost casual way "if you ever have the gumption to run across America…" which is pretty much like telling a bunch of non-astronauts that they should just get up the courage to apply to NASA. I'm back to the idea that this is all very inspiring and all very unrealistic in a lot of ways.

I shook his hand after his talk- one of the few audience members to have the audacity to do so. And his firm grip and good eye contact further belie his talk of being bashful. Dean Karnazes is also a businessman, and a good one. I mutter something about how inspirational he is before his handler whisks him away to the Greek Yogurt table at the Expo.

And he is inspirational, absolutely. The things he's done and seen are incredible to think about. I won't mirror his accomplishments anytime soon, but I appreciated his insight. In a very real way, runners are an odd little community. A community of individuals committed to the same individual pursuit. That's an interesting thing, isn't it?

But one thing really resonated with me from his talk. Almost casually, near the beginning, he captured what I like about running and what I have struggled with:

"Sometimes it's nice to get away and be in your own head for an hour."

# 30. "THE GREATEST REWARD FOR DOING IS THE OPPORTUNITY TO DO MORE." – DR. JONAS SALK

Day 30(!!!!!!)

A tiny bit more snow, and a whole lot more running. A half marathon today!

What the heck am I doing?! I sit here waiting for friends to pick us up – that would be Trent and his wife Cari. Cari is also running in the half-marathon, but Trent isn't crazy enough. Trent has a built in excuse because they have a youngster at home. It's the coldest day of the winter so far at 27 degrees. It's dark. Didn't I promise myself I wasn't going to run in the dark? It's snowy, and I'm not sure I have run below freezing since high school. Okay, some flag football in college was in the snow. Why would you run in below freezing temperatures?

I have hustled everything I'm taking into a series of bags, having abandoned my plan to have six upper layers, which consisted of

- Long sleeve tech shirt
- Plastic bag
- Short sleeve tech shirt
- Light Vest
- Light outer layer – running jacket
- Heavy outer layer (from goodwill) to discard

Yeah. I realized this was probably not going to work. I left the redundant vest and went with ONLY five layers, understanding that one layer would be tossed at the starting line and I'd have four – a light four layers, but four layers on my torso.

Bottom layers? I have three – running tights, shorts, and another throwaway layer. I'm definitely overthinking this, but I can't imagine anything that will spoil my day more than being miserably cold on the course.

So I pack all the other accoutrements, watch, gloves, another watch, FRD, heaphones, ipod, and layers to change into afterwards into bags, and as Trent and Cari arrive, throw everything in the car and we're off. What, no luggage?

Trent's Forerunner handles the ice easily, and an hour later Cari, Denise, and I get out of the car and head to Seattle Center, an hour early. We look like a lot like we might have slept in the street, wearing garbage bags and thick sweaters as outer layers. Photographers and police play the profiling game with us, "homeless or runner?" I can't speak for the police, but we pass four photographers before they ask if we'd like a shot. Denise and I pull up our garbage bag/sweater to reveal our bib numbers. Cari pulls down her pants. Well, her bib was pinned on her hip.

At the Seattle Center, we relax. I get a Peppermint Mocha. We use the bathroom. Uh, separately of course. Saying "we used the bathroom" – there's really no way to make that not sound awkward, is there?

There are hundreds of people milling about inside before the race, in various stages of relaxation. Most of them talk animatedly with one another, and some remind me of waiting to go running in the military. They stare into space. The annoying people jump about, loosening up. Well, I think it's annoying. One person has a yoga mat out. An actual yoga mat. Is he going to carry it when he runs?

At around ten minutes before the race starts, we go out into by the Space Needle where the race will begin. A mass of people crowds the starting line, but that's okay – the chip time doesn't start until we cross the mat. I kiss my wife, get my watches going – both sync, and we begin filing forward towards the starting line as the clock hits 7:30 am. It takes a few minutes to get to the start, and I'm occupied by taking off my outer layer as the crowd of runners starts presses forward. The ever-so-happy announcer blares through the speakers "you're looking good! You look great everyone! Here we go! You're looking good! You look great" she's insanely happy about the whole thing. I wince in pain at the volume.

And we're off.

Moving forward, stopping, starting, everyone tries to get enough space to run, and finally we do as the slinky-wave of runners expands. This lasts for the first half-mile. After that there is a bit of space, enough to run around the side if you want to. Which I do, because as has already been established, I'm a fool and I start too fast. If I ever get to the point where I can maintain this too-fast pace for a long time, I might be okay at this. But this is what us non-competitives have to deal with – a huge throng of runners moving in unison, trying to find their spot in an enormous line.

Along the way, a spectator yells at us: "POINT-ONE MILES!" Okay, that is funny.

I start out just behind the 2:30 pacer, holding their sign aloft. I pass them foolishly. The adrenaline boost I'm feeling is nice. Scott Douglas, an editor at Runner's World magazine, says: "In the first half of the race, don't be an idiot. In the second half, don't be a wimp!" I am not following his advice. Probably won't follow any part of it.

The crowd cruises along Fifth Avenue and we hit a bit more downhill as we pass the Seattle library. Some people are peeling back their layers – I can tell this because there are random hats and headbands strewn on the ground, things that fell. I can tell this because I see one person remove a hat and drop their glasses onto the ground. She doesn't see them fall, but a runner behind her does. That runner picks them up and runs after her, handing them back. Isn't that nice?

A gust hits us, blasting up from the Seattle waterfront to our right, eliciting a few yelps from the crowd.

In the first three miles I default to my performance instinct: "hey, I can finish sub-2:30!" It's still a major press of bodies along this stretch. Of course, soon after that nonsense I find myself slowing down. I feel it and try to pull back my pace, but have to stop halfway up the ramp over I-5. It's 23:00 into the course. I remind myself that isn't bad for me.

The sun starts peering over First Hill, illuminating the Seattle skyline.

In each of my prior races there is an interesting phenomenon – I usually end up running near someone with a similar pace. Usually it's a game of leapfrog as we alternatingly pass each other, walk, get passed, repeat. I think I've found my man at mile three, a forty-something guy with a yellow jacket, dripping sweat. We play leapfrog.

At mile four I'm snot-stained and wasted. Everyone passes me. Every young kid, every old person. Every person with a limp or a Chihuahua passes me. Such is the price of walking. It appears that the average half-marathoner has awesome stamina. They are all still running. You people are so awesome. Where are my walking peeps? The only people I am passing are the people standing in line at the porta-potties.

Will I end up as road kill somewhere on the course, a frozen slug?

But this is for me, right? That's difficult to remember when you're running with others. I started running for me, and I'm going to finish running for me.

Well played, everyone passing me. Some people can barely shuffle. Some people fly by.

I feel it in my calves already. Aha, a slight downhill. Gotta run this part.

We head into the tunnel at Interstate-90. I stop at the tables to get a bit of water. People whoop and yell in the tunnel, which reverberates off the walls and creates a din.

Both watches go along fine until we hit the tunnel. The Forerunner bonks out at this point. We come out of the tunnel and take a right, left, right left to loop back towards Seattle along the western edge of Lake Washington, an area called Leschi. I stop at a water break for Gatorade. The porta-potties are full with a line. Having to go while running is a real thing.

I take a moment to appreciate the beautiful houses as we run by. People stand in the cold to cheer us on. These are all view homes with their manicured hedges and sweeping views. They aren't sold by Re-Max. They're sold by Sotheby's. We all enjoy their spectacular views of Lake Washington, the city of Bellevue and the mountains in the distance. We pass by a small marina with sailboats.

And great cheers for the fans and the volunteers. So many people give of their time at these events to cheer runners on, to help us keep going. That's inspiring in itself.

Cymbals and cowbells greet me at mile five, which I get to in 55 minutes. I have to feel good about that. I realize I have run farther today than at any time in any run this month..! I'm having a great run so far, and I picked a heckuva day to do it. Whether it is the crowd and the adrenaline, I don't know, but I enjoy it.

One of my stated goals here was to experience the runner's high. Nope, nah, nothing so far this month, but you really don't get a runner's high at the short distances I've been running. You have to get to a point where you are exhausted for your body to roar back like that. The endorphins are a natural response to pain. I haven't had enough pain, I guess?

I stop for Gatorade again and scoot near the medical tent. You know, just in case.

The 2:30 pacer passes me.

From the bottom of Leschi, we cross into Madrona, by Madrona park, and we start climbing. And climbing. One street is so steep that most people stop to walk it. I am, obviously, part of "most people."

I hear the drums of a marching band. I love marching bands! We pass a group of ten drummers, Boom tikkatikkatikka Boom! Perradiddle whamadiddle Boom Boom!

Because I've run so many days in a row, this still feels like another run. It's a tough one, to be sure, but I'm hanging with it. I am pleasantly surprised at this.

Around six miles in, with only a tiny bit of cramping and soreness?

This feels like something I can do!

I hit the 10k marker at one hour and nine minutes. I hope someone here speaks Canadian because I'm not sure how far that is.

What's most impressive about the other runners isn't that I'm being passed by these youthful gazelles, the guys who have hardly broken a sweat or the women who look like they are trying to jazzercise their way to the finish line. The most impressive thing is that I'm being passed by people who outweigh me. I know how hard it is to lug my body along at my weight. How much tougher for them? I'm being passed by people far older than I am. They are out here doing it and they are kicking butt. It's getting harder for me at this point.

I got a good look at all of them because they all passed me, and I never caught up to them. Flaws and nonsense and all. Kudos to those brave ones today.

Earlier I said that this experience might be a lot like being "punched in the gut repeatedly" for thirteen miles.

I was way off. It's more like being punched in the sole of your foot for thirteen miles. Then your quadriceps, then every once in a while a punch to the back of your calf. Then a knock on the knee when you get used to the calf thing. My gut is fine.

It's a lot like being attacked by a gang of thugs whose sole intent is to attack your legs.

Or being attacked by the sport of running. As is everyone else is around me. A woman gyrates her shoulders with every step – that will hurt later. Another woman sounds like she has rocks for shoes – her footfall is so heavy it sounds painful. I run behind a gray-haired man who is probably 74 with "gizmo" embroidered on the back of his hat. His gait is terrible and he leans out too far. He left me in the dust too. A heavy set walker with saddle bags bigger than my hips. I couldn't catch her to save my life. Take a bow, lady! One guy was probably 6'3" and 270 pounds. A giant guy with plain cotton shorts, wavy hair, drenched in a plain cotton t-shirt at 27 degrees. He's keeping it crazy and killing it. All these brothers and sisters out here separately challenging the course for no other reason than to prove they can.

This run is absolutely breathtaking. As in, I can't seem to catch my breath.

It's somewhere around mile seven, and I am getting that very spent feeling. Somewhere along the way I accidentally stopped my Nike+ sportswatch, so when I hit it again the time kept going, but it's telling me my pace is 0'00" per mile. I don't think that's accurate. It's certainly not inspiring. Since the Forerunner couldn't take the tunnel, I have no idea what my pace is. Of course this means it is up to me and my legs.

It always has been.

An older gentleman shakes a cowbell at us in support. He's not running, he's just an athletic supporter. Speaking of which, my chafing issues so far are absolutely nonexistent. YAY. A little bit of a product called glide – applied twice this morning – has done the trick. This is a small thing but a major victory today. If you start chafing, your run can end painfully. I've got enough of that going right now, thanks.

A water break, I move to the side. At each water break there are volunteers handing out Gatorade and water, and the entire surface is icy from water freezing to the asphalt. On the other side of the tables there are cups strewn everywhere. I sip mine down and discard the cup, trying not to spill. Or fall. And wow, water is starting to taste good. It's a gourmet meal. Yum yum. Is there a touch of curry in this?

Okay, I might be a tad dehydrated. But the course starts downhill now, so I have to take advantage of that with some actual running. After every water break I feel refreshed, rejuvenated. A simple walk break does not have the same effect, but a water break feels fantastic. I pass mile eight, and we turn into the arboretum, a tree-lined road which is mostly downhill. I speed up.

It's clearly a second wind. I struggled from mile three to mile eight, but as I descend into the arboretum my speed picks up and I trot out a sub-eight-minute mile effortlessly. Another guy about my age keeps pace with me, or me him, and we pass dozens of runners, he on the left side of the road and I on the right. Running here is freedom, energy, difficult but so exhilarating.

We reach the bottom of the hill and start another climb up to the Interlaken trail. I stop for a walk break, still feeling good but tired again.

If you started reading this book expecting a 30-day descent into madness, well, I have to say I was with you. It's a bit daft to run for 30 days and decide halfway through to run four times farther the last day, just on a whim. But this is the culminating project of my madness. My transformation into cuckoo is complete here at mile nine. What else do I call this place where I run only to challenge myself, I have five miles left. What else do you call a run where I struggle for eight miles, and finish mile nine faster than any other mile I've run in this 30 day period?

At mile nine I have the unmistakable feeling that I WILL make it. And I feel so much better about it than before. I have about the equivalent of one of my daily runs left, and I am feeling it. If I woke up on any day this month feeling like I do now, I would probably not have made it.

Interlaken is a beautiful tree-lined bike trail between Lake Washington and Lake Union – as the name implies. It winds around the hillside with an overlook of "The Cut," the channel between the lakes.

The problem is that this trail winds around and around, flattens, and rises, flattens, and rises. This is a challenge, because I am discovering this for the first time and it seems interminable. "Another hill," I mutter. "yay."

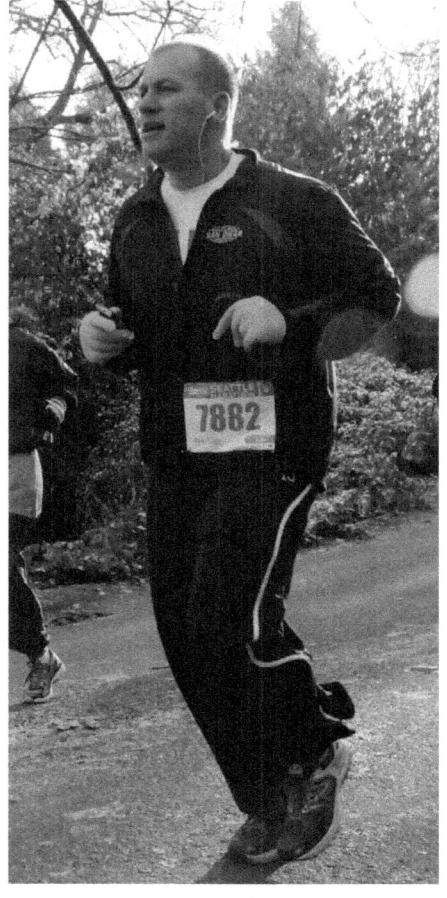

I'm gassed. But the course is the course, of course. After my second wind, I feel like it's taking everything I have to stay on it and not stop. But where would I stop and what would I do?

It's daunting. I walk, but I'm not angry, not like my last attempt at this. Somewhere along the way during this month I developed more of a tolerance for pain. I feel it, but it doesn't affect my mindset in the same way.

I guess what I'm saying is I'm not quite so much of a wimp as when I started.

I'm walking almost half of the time now, but the group around me seems to sense victory and surge forward. It's harder and harder to keep up, and all my pacer-buddies are long gone, except for a couple that stops at practically every porta-potty, passes me, and stops again. Except for a big Samoan with a camouflage hydration pack that looks to be struggling as I am. "Let's do this, big man," I say. He hears me about as well as I stay with him, which is to say "not so much." It's a solo struggle, and after a while everything else is just noise.

We turn away from the University of Washington and back towards Seattle, leaving the trail for a road. As I get slower and slower my hips start to tighten up. Gizmo passes me again for the last time.

A man holds up a dozen donuts. I can't even think about donuts, and I love donuts. It seems like a recipe for disaster. I know some people work out until they throw up, but there's no reason to tempt fate, is there? Ask me after the race, fella. Behind him it's another first aid station and blaring rap music. I derive a bit of bounce out of it, dance along and rally past that checkpoint, where I walk again. Oh goody, a hill. It was fun while it lasted.

As I stretch my way up the hill, I feel a twinge in my knee. Ouch. It's not serious. At least I think it isn't. I walk it off.

This is the part that will challenge me. This is the part where we will see what I am made of. The last three miles, after having run ten miles already. I'll find out what I'm made of. Has my training helped break down my bad attitude about running? Can I enjoy the rest of the run?

My back starts to tighten up.

My improved tolerance for pain serves me well. I soldier on, lamely. Why are there no medical tents in this part of the course? Why do I ask? Just wondering. In case it comes up. No reason.

The half-marathon sign says mile twenty-four. I'm eleven miles in! woof. My friend Cari catches up to me and we commiserate about our injuries so far. I am unable to hang with her either. She recedes into the distance in front of me, injuries and all.

Now the pain isn't the point. The point is finishing.

I'm alternating running fifty to one-hundred yards at a time now, and I have ladies running by me very slow talking to each other the entire time. Ugh.

Seattle opens up before us, and I see my goal in front of me. 30 days of running. And the Space Needle is the finish line. I don't have incredible insights on this run. The journey really is the destination, and I can't spare myself the luxury of waxing philosophic. I just want to conquer the distance, plain and simple, climb the mountain "because it's there." And then ask for oxygen.

That doesn't make the mountain easier. The hills of Seattle are grueling. Last hill? Nope. Okay, this must be the last hill! Nope.

I pass a man smoking from some fancy pipe or some kind of vaperphernalia. And an empty box by the side of the road labeled "lentils." Yeah, we're back in Seattle now.

A good jaunt down the off-ramp, down side streets back to Seattle Center. At mile twenty-five I am walking again, not even fast. It's almost a twenty-minute pace. I do curse now – I curse my dumbass training regimen. It gave me a slight tolerance for pain, but that's all I can say about it. I know I'm only scratching the surface of pain here in the grand scheme of things, but I am thankful that the pain I feel seems tolerable now.

People hold up their hand-crafted signs. My new favorite sign "You've done crazier things when drunk!" That is absolutely true, I tell the sign-holder as I pass. Another good one: "I don't do marathons. I do marathon runners." People are fun. The last water break, ambrosia again.

When you are totally spent, when there is nothing left of you but you must find strength, your mind searches frantically around for anything to get you across the finish line. And so I find my last burst of anything – I won't call it speed, that's inaccurate – my last burst of anything faster than a walk. I find the last vestige of what I have to use.

It's food. I think of having a pizza and it's easier somehow. My mind makes up a new mantra:

Pizza. Beer. Breakfast. Eggs. Sausage. Bacon. Bacon!

Like some reverse Maslow's hierarchy, my mind fixates on what it can understand: eating! If you can overeat in your mind, I need to join overeater's anonymous. I may need therapy after this, but I go with it. My mind thinks of every greasy thing it can and my body uses the fictional energy to speed me up. It gets me a half a mile further along, and that much is everything now.

Baconbaconbacon.

It doesn't last, of course, because the last quarter mile has another infernal HILL…!

*shakes fist at course designers*

Leave everything on the field? OKAY.

The last hill up to the stadium and the finish line. I find my buddy with the camouflage hydration pack struggling too and give him a word of encouragement. It's only a few hundred yards as we turn left to Seattle Center and enter the stadium, run across the field and through the finish line. I finish strong for no real reason other than the feeling of triumph. It feels alone, strangely. All the spectators are waiting for someone else, the cameramen are reloading, and the announcer is on break. It's silent as I pass, which suits me because I imagine the end of my life to be silent, and I'm past exhausted. A medal is placed on my neck, I grab a space blanket from people who don't seem to notice me, an energy bar, a bottle of water. I stagger inside to the recovery area. Everyone is so excited and happy around me, talking with each other. I'm just spent.

I am soaked through all layers. I pound the water bottle and crunch through the brick-hard energy bar. I have enough energy to chew it, but it's a struggle. I down a bottle of recovery drink inside, find my wife and Cari. I have nothing left to think, say, or do. I could go to sleep in the corner right now, I am that tired. I'm not in danger of losing consciousness, but if you asked me to say something intelligent you'd get little more than gibberish – and only after waiting for a few minutes.

I am finished.

# Race Results

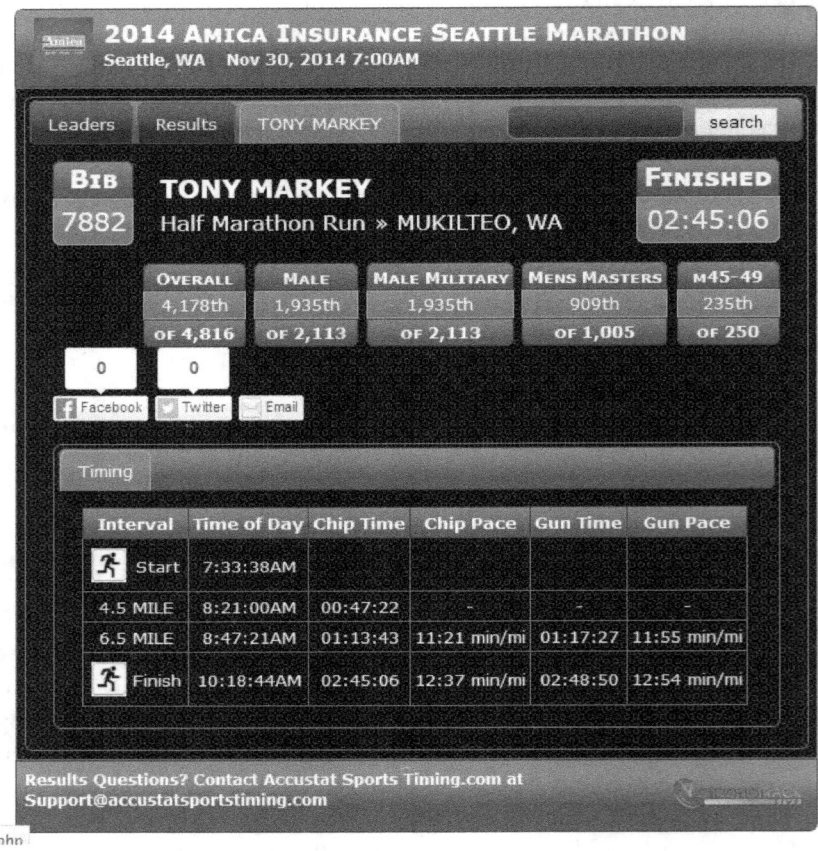

At home, I'm 238 pounds after the race.

# 31+. "YOU ARE NEVER TOO OLD TO SET ANOTHER GOAL OR DREAM A NEW DREAM" – C.S. LEWIS

Ow.

My legs are stiff. My joints and ligaments curse me. Strangely, I can walk. I'm surprised at that.

I am hungry as heck, though. I have that feeling that I can eat anything, I can't get full, and I'm still a bit dehydrated. I try to drink more water.

Bless my heart, I stank it up on the course, placing 235th out of 250 in my age group. That is abysmal, if you're keeping track of such things. But it's what I did. And it has value to me.

My journey has been was a wild ride. It's fascinating for me to reflect that when this experiment began I seriously doubted my ability to complete 30 days of running, not only mentally, but physically. I was sure that at some point the pain would be too great and I'd have to stop. More than a hundred years ago there were people who said that you couldn't ride in a car at 30 miles per hour. Surely you would suffocate. As it turns out, you can indeed ride in a car at 30 miles per hour. Someone risked life and limb to prove those naysayers wrong. Similarly, I have completed something I didn't really think I would be able to do, but which, in truth, was pretty simple.

I can indeed run for 30 minutes every day. In fact, not only was I able to, but I started to get a real "charge" out of doing so, somewhere about two-thirds of the way through. It's weird, but even the day after a half-marathon I feel like I can run – not fast, not painless, but I could run.

I'm still giving myself the day off, however. I mean, I still have some semblance of sanity left.

Once I had dealt with running and let go of my hatred of it, I could explore enjoying it. Running is a Rorschach test, where I draw conclusions based on mindset and pre-conception. I hope I have learned how to work at stopping this tendency of judging every run, of evaluating, of overanalyzing and trying to make everything mean something important.

I hated running because I was running with so much baggage, carrying everything along with me instead of trying to enjoy the moment.

Lessons! I did learn a few things that – if you were inclined – you might apply.

I had to disassociate myself from the outcome whenever possible. Faster, fitter, stronger? Try take that all out. It's surprisingly hard. Run without a danged watch sometimes. Run when the weather sucks – because who cares if you suck when it's snowing? Of course you suck. But that's not the point. Own the suckage.

Take whatever you can get. Work with what you have, and accept the outcome. The course is always unforgiving. How you perceive it can change.

Run in new places! This distracted me on some days, and it was wonderful when it did. Don't be afraid to stop and smell the roses – literally, if there are actual roses. Why not? You're not racing to your grave, are you? Are you worrying about your watch again?

Keep going. If you put one foot in front of the other, all the rest will come naturally. And if it doesn't, claim a victory anyway. For me being out there was a victory. Sucking but persevering was a victory. What is victory for you?

I also learned that other people are really strong. Stronger than me! But all we have is what we are, and that is enough for today.

I learned lessons every day. I learned on day twenty-six. I learned on day eight. I learned something about a lot of things, mostly about myself.

Am I a runner? The million dollar question. I balk at it, really. I like using phrases that are more neutral, like "Tony can be seen running" and "Tony runs often," rather than substituting in words like "avid" or "love." So it's an afterword that reads like a prologue, really. The lessons learned are my own. The running journey is your own. I can't make decisions for you; only for me, and I have to make that decision every day. Only you can take that excursion. There is no "completion." *The journey is the destination.*

Am I a runner? I might respond with:

"Well, I ran today. Maybe I'll run tomorrow too. What makes someone a runner?"

I love what running is – it's you. Running is whatever you make it. It's a tool that can help you reflect. It can be a kind of meditation, it can be a physical challenge, or a test of endurance. It is all those things. I love the gifts it brought me this month, unexpected ones. I hope you find things that bring you gifts too – even if they are sometimes crappy gifts.

Joseph Campbell described the meaning of life. I think it applies to running, and to what I have concluded in this 30-day experiment:

"Life has no meaning. Each of us has meaning and we bring it to life."

So I would say: Running has no meaning. Each of us has meaning and we bring it to running.

Cheers to all you other ~~runners~~ "people who can be seen running." May you find your meaning! I hope I see you on the road.

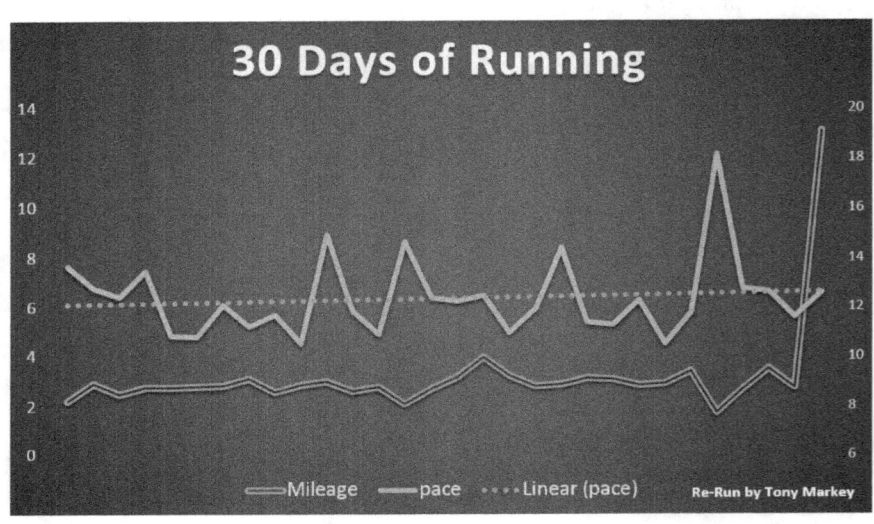

# A NOTE FROM THE AUTHOR

My Most Esteemed Reader,

If you're reading this, it means you got to the end of Re-Run. I'm sorry for that. I made it as long and entertaining as I could. All good things must end, sometimes with a 13(POINT ONE!!) mile run. I hope you enjoyed my journey at least as much as I did. Maybe a bit more than I did on those crap days. I hope that you can draw inspiration from my story in some way.

Except for concerts, I like feedback. Feel free to reach out to me at tonymarkey@hotmail.com, or check out my bloggity blog at http://www.tonymarkey.info

If you're so inclined, I'd love for you to review this book. Your feedback means that this might be shared with others via the internet because others like and favorite and tweet and Instagram and(insert newest web craze here) the book until everyone starts chanting my name and I am forced to come back out for a nifty encore where I shred the solo to "Roundabout" by YES on guitar, switch to bass to nail the far-out bassline, and sing a little harmony in the chorus as I finish the song on guitar. Woo! That would be awesome.

But regardless of whether or not that happens, I would still like to hear from you. It helps me know that you've connected with the material in some way.

So if my story was important to you, know that your story is important to me. Please refer back to wherever you bought this book to review it ☺

Thanks for picking up my work, and thanks in advance for sharing your opinion of it!

Best,

Tony Markey

# ABOUT THE AUTHOR

Tony Markey is a runner. Haha, just kidding. He's a hack. An absolute running hack. Not in a "life hack" way, but more like in a "hey slow guy, you suck!" way. He's an old fat guy that hopes that he doesn't have to be fat and slow forever. Still, he's not getting any younger. And he shares his collected wisdom so others can follow in his footsteps. Only not exactly in his footsteps, because that would take forever. Like, figuratively in his footsteps. Or like, in front of his footsteps.

Tony is a humorist, author, banjo player, father, and part-time geek. His vocational background mirrors the diversity of his hobbies, and he has worked, both successfully and with great tolerance for masochism in many industries, from retail to insurance to healthcare, from sales to analysis to management. He holds a Master's in Business Administration, if you must know, but he has pursued graduate work in Theater. He's either brilliant or terribly confused is what I'm trying to say. I mean he is trying to say. He is an expert at talking about himself in the third person.

Tony lives near Seattle with his wonderful wife and three amazing kids, one of which tolerates him. They take turns.